# KEEP YOUR

*wits*

# ABOUT YOU

# KEEP YOUR *wits* ABOUT YOU

---

## THE SCIENCE OF BRAIN MAINTENANCE AS YOU AGE

---

Vonetta M. Dotson, PhD

 **AMERICAN PSYCHOLOGICAL ASSOCIATION**

Published by
American Psychological Association
750 First Street, NE
Washington, DC 20002
https://www.apa.org

Order Department
https://www.apa.org/pubs/books
order@apa.org

In the U.K., Europe, Africa, and the Middle East, copies may be ordered from Eurospan
https://www.eurospanbookstore.com/apa
info@eurospangroup.com

Typeset in Sabon by Circle Graphics, Inc., Reisterstown, MD

Printer: Sheridan Books, Chelsea, MI
Cover Designer: Mark Karis

Library of Congress Cataloging-in-Publication Data

Names: Dotson, Vonetta M., author.
Title: Keep your wits about you : the science of brain maintenance as you age / Vonetta M. Dotson.
Description: Washington, DC : American Psychological Association, [2022] | Includes bibliographical references and index. | Summary: "This book provides science-based facts and practical tools to help readers develop healthy lifestyles to optimize their cognitive abilities, mental health, and physical functioning at any age"--Provided by publisher.
Identifiers: LCCN 2021047281 (print) | LCCN 2021047282 (ebook) | ISBN 9781433832895 (paperback) | ISBN 9781433832901 (ebook)
Subjects: LCSH: Older people--Mental health. | Cognitive neuroscience. | Mental health--Nutritional aspects. | Mental health--Physiological aspects.
Classification: LCC RC451.4.A5 D68 2022 (print) | LCC RC451.4.A5 (ebook) | DDC 618.97/689--dc23/eng/20211102
LC record available at https://lccn.loc.gov/2021047281
LC ebook record available at https://lccn.loc.gov/2021047282

https://doi.org/10.1037/0000283-000

Printed in the United States of America

10 9 8 7 6 5 4 3 2 1

To my parents, for instilling a love of learning in me
and always believing in me, and to my husband,
for helping me believe in myself.

# CONTENTS

# PREFACE

There is nothing I find more rewarding in my professional life than sharing my passion with the world. My passion is the brain. I am fascinated by how our brains shape, and are shaped by, the way we behave. I remember when I first fell in love with the brain. When I was in my junior year of college, I had my first experience learning about this incredible organ in a physiological psychology class. What captivated me the most was learning about the link between the brain and psychological conditions such as depression, which many people think of as being "mental" and not "physical." This realization that the mind and body are inextricably intertwined sealed my fate: I knew I had to pursue a career that focuses on how the brain influences behavior, from remembering a song to moving across a room. This passion led me to become a neuropsychologist.

I am a scientist–practitioner, which means I have dual expertise in conducting neuropsychological research and in providing clinical services. It also means that my clinical services are grounded in the latest scientific evidence. I have taken the same science-based approach in writing this book. In fact, the science-based recommendations I have given my clients over the past 20 years inspired me to write this book. I found myself wishing I had a resource to give my clients that not only summarizes what science tells us about how lifestyle and behavior affects our brain but also gives practical guidance for how to incorporate healthy behaviors into daily life. I wanted the resource to be informative, comprehensive, engaging, and brief. Finding no options that fit my criteria, I decided to create the resource I wanted my clients to have. In doing so, it has been my pleasure to do what I find most fulfilling—sharing my passion about brain health.

This book will give you knowledge and practical tools to set healthy habits that promote a healthy brain. Science tells us that when our brains are healthy, we are more likely to stay mentally sharp throughout our lives and less likely to develop conditions such as Alzheimer's disease and depression. To be clear, there is no magic bullet when it comes to brain health. Developing and maintaining a healthy brain requires a commitment to long-term habits that give you the best shot at living well, aging well, and avoiding the memory loss, cognitive decline, and other complications that arise when the brain is not healthy. Beware the books, websites, or commercial products that claim to have a quick fix or guaranteed method for boosting your memory or preventing dementia.

If you are reading this book, you are already taking a big step toward living life to the fullest. This is important regardless of how old you are. Aging well requires living well throughout our lives, so we must nurture and protect our brain at every age. Because this journey to a healthier brain is a lifelong process, remember to take it one step at a time. Change doesn't happen overnight, and habits don't develop overnight. But the effort is worthwhile! I am thrilled that you have decided to include me in your journey. I hope this book motivates you and empowers you to live a brain-healthy life.

# ACKNOWLEDGMENTS

My career has been shaped by many teachers, mentors, research collaborators, and colleagues who have enlightened, inspired, and challenged me. There are too many to name, but I would like to give a collective thank you to the brilliant people who have crossed my path and contributed to my career over the years. I would not be where I am without them. I especially want to thank Dr. Michael Marsiske, for guiding and mentoring me through graduate school and beyond, and Dr. Glenn Smith, for being my consummate advocate, mentor, and friend. I also want to acknowledge my current and previous graduate students and postdoctoral fellows. Like a proud parent, I am honored to have them as my academic children. They have affected my career as much as I have affected theirs.

I enjoyed interviewing a variety of researchers, students, and other people in my personal and professional life to illustrate different points in this book. I thank them for their time and contribution to bringing this book to life. I also thank the community of scientists worldwide whose research forms the basis of this book.

This book also would not have been possible were it not for a fateful Uber ride where I met my writing coach, Timothy Pratt. He helped me transform my writing from a manuscript only other researchers or health professionals would enjoy to an accessible book for all people. I cannot thank him enough for his guidance and support during the writing of this book.

Finally, I would like to thank my husband, my parents, and all of my friends and family who have encouraged and supported me throughout my career. They are my biggest cheerleaders and source of strength. To quote Maya Angelou, "I sustain myself with the love of family."

# KEEP YOUR
## *wits*
# ABOUT YOU

# INTRODUCTION

"Is there a cure for Alzheimer's disease?" "What can I do about losing my memory as I get older?" "How can I keep my mind sharp in retirement?" These are questions I hear on a regular basis from my clients. As a neuropsychologist who specializes in aging, I know that there currently is no cure for Alzheimer's disease. But I also know there is a large body of research showing that we *can* at least reduce our risk for Alzheimer's disease, and improve our memory and other cognitive abilities as we get older, by adopting healthy behaviors that boost the health of our brains. And I know that what we do throughout our life sets the course for how we age, so achieving and maintaining a healthy brain is a lifelong process.

This book is a science-based guide to maximizing your brain health throughout your life. On the basis of more than 20 years of professional experience—as a researcher, clinician, and teacher—since I began my graduate studies, I share with you expert recommendations for how to achieve and maintain the healthiest brain possible. You will learn how the health of your brain is linked to your memory and cognitive abilities, your mood, and other aspects of health. I also offer practical suggestions for how to make lifestyle changes that can benefit your brain.

## WHO SHOULD READ THIS BOOK?

The short answer to this question is—everyone! This book can benefit you if you're young or in your senior years, if you're at the peak of your cognitive skills or you're starting to experience memory loss, and if you're interested in brain health for yourself or for a loved one. As you will learn in the coming chapters, what you do at every stage of your life matters. Because my expertise is in later life, the examples I share from my clinical experiences are from clients in their 50s and older. I'm aware that midlife and later is the time when most people start to worry about their brain health, so I have made it a point to speak to issues relevant to the later stages of life. To be clear, though, the recommendations I will give you apply to people of all ages. Research tells us that you are more likely to age well if you start to adopt brain-healthy behaviors earlier in life, but you can still get some benefits if you start working on your brain health later in life.

## WHAT SHOULD YOU EXPECT?

This book focuses on the lifestyle behaviors that scientists have found to be most closely linked to brain health. These include getting enough physical, mental, and social activity; keeping good dietary patterns; getting enough high-quality sleep; and treating physical and mental health conditions. In the first chapter, I give an overview of why brain health is important and what you can do to achieve a healthier brain. I also provide some guidance about when to seek professional help and how to interpret information about brain health from different sources. Each of the six chapters that follow focuses on specific brain-healthy behaviors.

In each of these chapters, in the first section I outline what science tells us, and in the second section I dive into recommendations for making these behaviors a part of your life. In the third section I provide resources, mostly online, and suggested readings if you would like to learn more about topics we cover in the chapter. Some of the chapters include worksheets that you can use to brainstorm ideas or keep track of your progress. In the last chapter, I summarize what you've learned and offer some final tips for getting started and staying the course. All of the chapters include a list of references at the end so that, if you're interested, you can read the original research articles that provide the scientific basis of the chapter.

## HOW SHOULD YOU USE THIS BOOK?

My goal is that, after reading this book, you will have a better understanding of what science tells us about maintaining a healthy brain, you will be motivated to make changes to your lifestyle to improve your brain health, and you will have a blueprint for how to get started on your journey. Remember that it is indeed a journey. As I discuss in the last chapter, it is important to keep your motivation high by setting realistic goals instead of lofty ones. To set realistic goals, you will need to consider your own circumstances and resources. I encourage you to take time to reflect on what you've learned at the end of each chapter and to think about how you can take a step in a healthy direction within the context of your life. Use this book as a guide and as an inspiration to set personal goals.

This book is not intended to replace personalized care from a psychologist, physician, or other professional. If you have concerns about memory loss and cognitive decline, mental health, or other medical concerns, I encourage you to see a health care provider. In Chapter 1, I provide suggestions for when you might need to see a health care provider about memory loss and cognitive decline. Some of the other chapters describe warning signs for when you might need to see a professional for help (e.g., in Chapter 6,

I describe signs of a sleep disorder that might warrant a visit to a sleep specialist). You might even discuss the recommendations from this book with your health care provider and ask for their feedback about how to tailor the recommendations to your needs. Use this book as a resource in your journey to a healthier brain and a complement to your personal health care.

# CHAPTER 1

# WHAT IS A HEALTHY BRAIN, AND HOW CAN WE KEEP IT THAT WAY?

A 55-year-old woman came to my clinic, concerned about her memory. An elementary school teacher for nearly 30 years, she was used to remembering names, faces, and conversations without any problems. But now there were many times when a fellow teacher, family member, or friend referred to a conversation from the past that she did not remember. She would fake recalling the conversation, but she was convinced other people could see through her charade. She also noticed that she was misplacing objects, such as her keys and her reading glasses, more often than usual. Despite her concerns, her husband, who also came to the evaluation, had not noticed any changes in her memory.

I am a neuropsychologist, which means I specialize in how the brain is involved in our thoughts, emotions, and behavior. My clients come to me for an assessment of strengths and weaknesses in their memory, attention, and other cognitive abilities. I also evaluate their emotional functioning to determine whether they have a psychological disorder such as depression or anxiety.

My evaluation includes an interview with the client and a family member so that I can learn more about their concerns; medical and psychological history; and background information, such as education and work history. I then give the client a variety of standardized memory and cognitive tests, most using a paper and pencil, and a few that are done on a computer. Whenever possible, I gather medical records or talk to one or more of the client's physicians for more detailed medical information.

Then comes my favorite part: putting together all of this information like pieces of a jigsaw puzzle to get a picture of how the client's brain is functioning. How does this help the person with concerns about their memory? For one, my evaluation, along with other medical information, can help reveal a neurological diagnosis, such as Alzheimer's disease, or a psychological diagnosis, such as depression. This is an important first step toward seeking treatment. If people already have a diagnosis from their physician—say, Parkinson's disease or stroke—I can shine a light on how their medical condition is affecting their cognitive abilities and their day-to-day functioning. This allows the person and their family to make important decisions. Can they continue to work? Is it safe for them to drive? Should someone help them manage their money or medical care?

I gave the 55-year-old woman who came in to see me an evaluation similar to what I just described. It turned out that her memory was perfectly fine, as were her other abilities. She is what we neuropsychologists sometimes call the "worried well." These are people who become concerned about a possible serious issue when they notice slight changes in their memory or other cognitive skills in everyday life, but testing shows their brains have no serious, underlying problems. In many cases, the "worried well" have short-term stressors or medical issues that lead to small, temporary changes in how they function. I discuss in more detail when you should be concerned about your memory and other cognitive skills later in this chapter.

Another client who came to my clinic had different results. Her son and daughter-in-law asked me to evaluate her because they were very worried. Not only was this 74-year-old woman forgetting conversations and misplacing items—just like my first client—but she also was forgetting the names of family members, getting lost in familiar places, and confusing her medications.

Her family described a gradual decline in functioning over the previous 4 years, leading to the dramatic problems that prompted them to seek an evaluation. They mentioned a disturbing incident: The client walked out of the house without telling anyone, wandered to a store several miles away, and appeared so confused that the store manager looked through their phone for an emergency contact to call. As you might imagine, this was a striking change from her high level of functioning earlier in life. In fact, she had worked in health care for decades!

As I evaluated her, she was very pleasant and friendly. She appeared somewhat frail, and she walked slowly. She repeated the same information to me over and over, seemingly unaware that she had already said the same thing. She even forgot who I was after taking a bathroom break. Sometimes she responded to my questions with completely irrelevant information. She struggled when I tested her memory and other cognitive abilities. Ultimately, I diagnosed her with Alzheimer's disease.

These are two very different clients, whose neuropsychological evaluations led to different results. But in both situations a key part of my recommendations was exactly the same: Get more physical activity, stay socially connected, keep your mind engaged, and eat a healthy diet. Why would I give the same advice to someone whose mind is still sharp as I would to someone who has Alzheimer's disease? Because science tells us that the healthy behaviors I recommended are the most powerful tools we have to maintain healthy brains throughout our lives. In fact, people who practice those behaviors tend to have not only sharper minds but also better moods, and they are less likely to develop cognitive impairment, Alzheimer's disease, or other types of dementia as they age. This book will give you the science-based tools to help you achieve and maintain a brain-healthy lifestyle.

Some background information about the brain and about science will help you get the most out of this book. In this first chapter, I explain why brain health is important, what the consequences might be when your brain isn't healthy, and when you should seek professional help for memory loss and cognitive decline. Because scientific research forms the basis of this book, I also provide guidance here on how to interpret scientific research and how to sift through information about science in the media.

## WHAT IS A HEALTHY BRAIN?

Today I went to the news tab in Google and searched for "healthy brain." I found more than 100 matches published within the past month! Article titles ranged from "7 Foundations for a Healthy Brain" and "How to Eat for a Healthy Brain," to "6 Habits of Super Learners" and "Fish Oil Believed to Be a Liquid Gold Against Mood Disorders." Brain health is clearly a hot topic.

Why the intense interest in information about the brain? People are living longer: According to the Centers for Disease Control and Prevention, life expectancy in the United States has risen from a mere 47.3 years in 1900 to 78.6 years in 2017 (Devitt, 2018)! With that longer life span comes a higher risk of different medical conditions, including Alzheimer's disease, which is the most common cause of dementia. Because there is not yet a cure for Alzheimer's disease, many people are turning to nonpharmacological strategies to reduce their risk of developing the condition by maintaining a healthy brain.

This focus on the brain is warranted. Your brain is one of the most vital organs in your body. It is essential to every aspect of your life—each action you take, and each thought you have is a sign of your brain at work. The brain also supports your basic senses, such as vision and hearing, and orchestrates vital functions in your body, such as blood pressure and breathing. No wonder it is so important to protect and maintain a healthy brain!

A healthy brain is one that has the blood flow it needs to perform at peak level. This means that the brain's structure and the brain's function must be maintained as much as possible throughout your life. When I talk about *brain structure*, I am talking about attributes such as overall brain size or the size of different regions of the brain, such as the hippocampus, a region crucial for memory. *Brain function*, on the other hand, is the actual inner workings of the brain as it controls the activities of the body. As you go about living your life, behind the scenes billions of nerve cells called *neurons* are hard at work in your brain. These neurons send information to each other and to the rest of the body to make it possible for you to live, move, act, and think. Without neurons sending information to each other, you couldn't walk, talk, play an instrument, or solve a math problem. You couldn't even be alive!

## WHAT HAPPENS WHEN THE BRAIN ISN'T HEALTHY?

What is the first thing that comes to mind when you hear the term "brain disorder"? My guess is you thought of Alzheimer's disease. It seems that everyone is worried about Alzheimer's. Many of us have witnessed the memory decline, personality changes, and difficulty managing everyday tasks that are the telltale signs of this disease.

You are not alone if you are concerned about the health of your brain as you grow older. The AARP conducted a survey in 2015 to gauge how important brain health is to people over the age of 40 (Skufca, 2015). Three quarters of the people who responded were concerned about their brain health declining in the future. Another survey—this one from the National Council on Aging—found that in people over age 60, memory loss is the second most common concern, right behind physical health ("Health or Finances?," 2015).

Alzheimer's disease is the most common type of "dementia," which is an umbrella term for a variety of conditions that lead to a decline in cognitive functioning and interfere with a person's ability to perform everyday tasks such as driving, managing money, and basic self-care. All of these changes reflect problems with how the brain is functioning. Even though the risk of dementia increases with age, it stems not from the normal process of aging but rather from damage to brain cells. However, dementia is only one consequence of brain dysfunction. Your ability to move, your memory and cognitive skills, and even your mood are all affected by the health of your brain.

As a neuropsychologist, I wear many different hats. One of them is brain researcher. Over the past 20 years, I have studied the connections among the brain, cognitive functioning, and depression. My work focuses mostly on older adults. I am intrigued by the way the brain changes over the course of our life and how that affects so many aspects of our health and behavior. Early in my career, I studied what happens when something goes wrong in the brain: Depression, dementia, Parkinson's disease, and a host of other conditions can arise. My research goal was to help us understand what goes wrong in the brain so that we can then figure out how to make things right.

I have learned so much from this research! For example, my studies have shown that changes in brain structure and in brain function are closely connected to changes in mood (e.g., Dotson et al., 2021; McLaren et al., 2017; Szymkowicz et al., 2016). Even more fascinating is the fact that, as we get older, the connection between brain and mood gets even stronger. In other words, the brain changes researchers have pinpointed in people who are depressed are even more pronounced in older adults. My research also has shown that the link among brain changes, depression, and cognitive problems is not the same for everyone (e.g., Dotson, 2017; Dotson et al., 2018; Michalak et al., 2020). In fact, behavior that helps keep your brain healthy seems to provide a buffer against some of the cognitive difficulties, such as poor attention and slower mental speed, that often accompany depression. This highlights why such behaviors are so important!

## WHAT CAN YOU DO WHEN YOUR BRAIN ISN'T HEALTHY?

As I conducted this "what goes wrong" research I just mentioned, I became more and more interested in figuring out what we can do when things go wrong. I am keenly interested in the following three questions: (a) Can we prevent at least some of the disorders caused by brain dysfunction? (b) Can we slow down the progression of conditions such as dementia that ravage the brain? (c) And, most important to me, can healthy behaviors throughout our life positively affect the health of our brain as we age? These are the questions that drive my research now. My biggest goal is to understand what we can do throughout our lives to achieve and keep a healthy brain. By doing this, we can boost our cognitive skills, our mood, our physical functioning, and much more.

There are many studies from lots of different researchers that point to the same fact: The answer to my big three questions is a resounding *yes*! Healthy behavior throughout your life can benefit your brain. And, as a result, it is possible to prevent, delay, or slow down some brain diseases. How empowering is it to know that each and every one of us can make choices that lower our risk for developing memory issues, depression, Alzheimer's disease, and many other problems with our brains!

Let's be clear about an important point: Achieving and keeping a healthy brain takes work and a long-term commitment. Despite claims you might hear about "14 days to a better brain" or "brain pill enhancements," the truth is that you cannot truly boost your brain by completing a short-term training program or taking a pill. Instead, make a lifestyle change that includes as many of the healthy behaviors that science has shown to benefit your brain as you can.

What are those healthy behaviors? The big three—the ones that have the most scientific evidence—are physical activity, cognitive activity, and social activity. People who exercise regularly, keep their mind active by challenging it, and maintain social connections tend to have healthier brains. Studies have shown that people who adopt these behaviors early in life are more likely to maintain a healthy brain as they age. But even if you begin later in life, you still get a benefit, so it is never too late to start!

The health of your brain is also affected by your diet, your sleep habits, and different medical conditions—especially ones that affect your heart—and some psychological disorders. Each of these can also affect the other. For example, a high-fat diet can put you at risk for heart disease, which in turn raises your risk for depression. And in some people, one symptom of depression is difficulty sleeping, which has been linked to a higher risk of heart disease. So, a vicious cycle can develop. The good news is that when you live a brain-healthy lifestyle—which is also a heart-healthy lifestyle—you can interrupt that vicious cycle and have a happier, more fulfilling life.

I am working on this chapter during the COVID-19 pandemic. As I am sure you have experienced, this time of uncertainty created very real challenges to any type of normal routine. Combine this with all of the stressors to our own health and that of our loved ones, social isolation, and financial concerns, and it's no wonder that mental health is the focus of many news articles and blog posts published during the pandemic. I have come across suggestions for maintaining mental health during the COVID-19 outbreak that echo what we know about brain health in general. For example, *Psychology Today* posted a story on May 6, 2020, called "7 Ways to Promote Brain Health During a Pandemic" (Randolph, 2020). A board-certified clinical neuropsychologist offered the following seven tips:

1. Stay physically active.
2. Maintain a structured schedule.
3. Stay mentally engaged.
4. Maintain physical, not necessarily social, distancing.
5. Mobilize your stress management strategies.
6. Eat as well as possible.
7. Sleep in the Goldilocks zone (i.e., maintain a consistent sleep schedule).

Do you notice the similarities in that list and in the brain-healthy behaviors I just mentioned? These behaviors are helpful not only in the long term; they can enhance your well-being in the short term as well. Again, this is not to say that these are a quick fix. Understand that you can benefit from engaging in these behaviors in the short term, but you will need to incorporate them into your life on a regular basis to realize the long-term benefits.

## WHEN TO SEEK HELP FOR MEMORY LOSS AND COGNITIVE DECLINE

A healthy lifestyle can help us lower our risk for cognitive problems throughout our life. But we have to be realistic that the most we can do is *reduce* our risk; we cannot be certain that we will *eliminate* all risk. Throughout our life, a variety of injuries; illnesses; infections; and substances, such as medications, illicit drugs, and environmental toxins, can cause problems with memory and cognitive functioning. And as we get older, it is common for certain types of memory and cognitive skills to decline. For example, we might become more forgetful, find it more challenging to multitask, or have mild difficulty paying attention. When should you be concerned that you or a loved one might have something serious going on that is affecting memory, attention, or other cognitive skills?

When it comes to any health concern, whether it be about cognitive functioning, physical health, or mental health, my general advice is to talk to your doctor if you are worried. If you are in your 60s or older, I recommend you see a *geriatrician*, a doctor who specializes in treating older adults. It is better to ask than to ignore changes in how you're feeling or functioning. But there are specific situations that suggest getting your cognitive skills checked out would be a good idea.

Regardless of your age, talk to your doctor if you notice changes in your cognitive functioning after a head injury, a seizure, or another medical condition that affects your brain. Another important sign is when you notice that memory loss, attention problems, or other cognitive difficulties make it hard for you to carry out your usual daily activities, such as driving, functioning at work or school, cooking, or shopping. This is especially important as we get older, because trouble performing daily activities is one of the criteria for Alzheimer's disease and other types of dementia.

Many older adults worry about their memory. For example, my 55-year-old "worried well" client is a classic example of someone having normal age-related forgetfulness because she had concerns about her memory, but testing showed that she was in the range I would expect for her age. It was still worthwhile for her to get evaluated because she felt distressed by the changes she was seeing, so the evaluation helped ease her mind. This is important because stress and anxiety can interfere with cognitive functioning. On top of that, it can be very helpful as you get older to get a neuropsychological evaluation to set a *baseline*: Once you are evaluated and have a summary of your test scores, those scores can be used as a basis for comparison if you start to notice more significant problems down the road and have another evaluation. This allows the neuropsychologist to chart *changes* in your functioning, which can give us much more information than seeing you on one occasion.

Not everyone experiences normal age-related forgetfulness to the same degree; in fact, some people maintain memory and other cognitive skills into their 70s, 80s, and beyond. But other people have problems that are cause for concern, problems that are not a part of normal aging. For example, it is not normal to get lost in familiar places, have trouble following instructions, or become confused about where you are or what year or month it is. Think of the significant problems my client with Alzheimer's disease had, such as wandering away from home. These are concerning signs that should prompt you to talk to your doctor and request a neuropsychological evaluation. I also suggest talking to your doctor if you notice a very sudden drop in your memory and cognitive functioning from one week or one month to the next, because normal age-related decline is usually gradual rather than abrupt.

I specifically suggest that you ask your doctor for a referral to a neuropsychologist because neuropsychologists specialize in cognitive testing and have the expertise to understand how the brain relates to different aspects of behavior, such as cognitive functioning and emotion. Medicare pays for neuropsychological evaluations, and many other insurance providers provide at least partial coverage for neuropsychological services. There are other health care providers whose expertise overlaps with neuropsychologists, such as neurologists, psychiatrists, and psychologists with other specialties, but these other specialists are less likely to have the combination of expertise in cognitive testing plus expertise in brain functioning. Most of the clients who come to see me have a neurologist or psychiatrist as well, and often it is one of those specialists who refers them to me. The best care is integrated care, so in the ideal situation your neuropsychologist will be in communication with your other health care providers to make sure everyone is informed and on the same page about your health.

When in doubt, get checked out. In some cases, it might be appropriate for you to have a brief screening evaluation. This might involve a 30-minute interview with a neuropsychologist followed by 20 to 30 minutes of cognitive testing to get a quick snapshot of your functioning. If you do well on the screening, that might be all you need. If the screening picks up on any possible problems, you can then receive a more thorough evaluation. A full neuropsychological evaluation usually involves a thorough interview, usually lasting from 60 to 90 minutes, and multiple hours of cognitive testing depending on the condition for which you're being evaluated. Dementia evaluations, such as the ones I give to most of my clients, usually involve 2 to 3 hours of cognitive testing. On the other hand, evaluations for attention-deficit/hyperactivity disorder or learning disorders often involve a full day (6–7 hours), or even 2 days, of testing. When you schedule an appointment, make sure to ask how long the evaluation will last and how you should prepare for your appointment.

I have noticed more and more websites popping up that offer memory testing or cognitive testing that you can give yourself at home. I would not recommend at-home cognitive testing. Your brain health is part of your overall health, so you should trust it to a licensed health care provider. In the same way that you would not give yourself a blood test and try to decipher the results to see if you have high cholesterol or diabetes, you should not try to do your own assessment of cognitive functioning.

Regardless of the results of a neuropsychological evaluation for you or your loved one, chances are the neuropsychologist will recommend many of the brain-healthy behaviors you will learn about in this book. Science tells us that incorporating these behaviors into our lives benefits us before and after we experience cognitive decline.

## THE TIME TO START IS NOW!

In my work, clients and their families often ask if it's too late to do anything to help memory, especially if the client already has dementia. When I teach undergraduates, my students have a completely different mindset: They often exclaim that they never even considered the brain as needing to be healthy. If we took these two perspectives to be true, then only middle-aged people would need to think about brain health because we don't need to worry about it early in life and our brains can't be changed in old age. But this could not be further from the truth! Remember that your brain is one of your most vital organs. It needs to be healthy throughout your entire life, from cradle to grave. And because we know that the brain is able to rewire and develop new cells in your older years, and even in people who have a brain disease, it is never too late to achieve a healthier brain!

Clients who come to see me for a neuropsychological assessment come back for a second appointment to get feedback regarding my evaluation. This is when I talk to the client and their family about what they can do to achieve a better quality of life. A huge part of that is improving brain health. I give my clients specific recommendations to address any diagnosis or symptoms they have, and I try to kick-start their motivation to bring healthier behaviors into their life. In fact, this part of my work as a neuropsychologist is what prompted me to write this book! Instead of relying on one conversation in a 60-minute feedback session, I want my clients—and everyone interested in bettering their lives—to have a guide for their journey toward healthier brains.

When I held a feedback session with my 74-year-old client with dementia, her son and daughter-in-law attended. Family involvement is especially important when the client has memory impairment because I cannot expect the client to remember all my recommendations. I explained to this client and her family the importance of certain behaviors for brain health. I emphasized the need for her to exercise as much as possible, keep her mind engaged, build her social network, and have a good diet. Her family immediately began brainstorming about how to make these activities a regular part of her week. What thrilled me was that most of their ideas involved all of them doing things together as a family, such as taking walks together, playing games that would stimulate her mind, and cooking together. This meant that as the 74-year-old woman was improving her brain health to slow down her dementia, her middle-age family members, and even her teenage grandchildren, were going to be improving their brain health, too!

There is no time limit on achieving a healthy brain. Whether you're in your 20s, your 50s, or your 80s, the time to start is now! The question is, how do you make and maintain changes in your lifestyle that will promote your health?

I posed this question to Tina Williamson, an Emory University–certified health and wellness coach who works with my company, CerebroFit Integrated Brain Health. CerebroFit helps people put into action all of the brain-healthy behavior I am recommending in this book by offering online and in-person services, such as neuropsychological assessment, personal training, nutrition services, psychotherapy, and health and wellness coaching with Tina. As a health and wellness coach, Tina specializes in helping people find motivation and overcome obstacles in pursuit of health goals. She has had a front-row seat to transformations in her clients and in students who have taken her group fitness classes over the past 30 years. She has helped people break free from chronic illnesses such as obesity, diabetes, and autoimmune disorders by changing their lifestyle habits and behaviors.

The long and short of Tina's answer to my question was this: "For sustained change to become a lifestyle, one must show up mentally and physically to craft their own personal goals and commit to take realistic action steps." Let's break down this sage advice.

Tina mentioned sustained change becoming a lifestyle. This echoes my earlier point that health—and, in the case of this book, brain health—does not happen overnight. Expect to make changes in your behavior that become habits, which lead to a brain-healthy lifestyle.

An important part of Tina's advice is "One must show up mentally and physically." She explained that after 30-plus years of teaching the "how to get fit, stay fit, and get fitter philosophy in schools and gyms," she realized that to truly help people discover how to live a healthier life, one must "go beyond physical intelligence and include the goals of mental awareness and spiritual (or social) understanding." Body, mind, and spirit are connected. Making sustained lifestyle changes requires involving all three.

Tina advises her clients to "craft their own personal goals and commit to taking realistic action steps." In this book I offer practical advice for incorporating brain-healthy behaviors into your life, but the key to your success is setting specific goals for yourself and taking steps toward the goals that are realistic for you. The process will not look exactly the same for each of us. Tina also emphasized that motivation is good and necessary, but it is never enough. Accountability is the key. For some people, a health coach such as Tina is a great way to be held accountable to the goals they set. If hiring a health coach is not an option for you, think of someone else in your life who will hold you accountable, and include them as you embark on your lifestyle changes.

As you make changes to promote your brain health, don't hesitate to seek help from family members, friends, or professionals as needed. In fact, having a partner such as a workout buddy can be crucial to maintaining new habits. In Tina's experience, the most common obstacle to changing behavior is the inability or unwillingness to admit we need help, which blocks us from growth and improvement. "My experience is that folks who have the courage to be vulnerable have the strength to change," she said.

Tina made a statement that resonated with me because it mirrors my own motivation, as a neuropsychologist, in writing this book. She said her greatest satisfaction as a health and wellness coach is "the indescribable joy of watching someone transform their lives through self-discovery and appropriate action—simply put, to witness a fellow human being freed from the obstacles that bind them!"

We all have obstacles—financial, emotional, and physical, for example—to consistently adopting behaviors that would improve the health of our brains. But with a foundation of sound scientific knowledge and practical suggestions, my hope is that you will find your motivation and seek out the accountability you need to transform your life.

## TAKE YOUR CUES FROM LEGITIMATE SOURCES

The purpose of this book is to give you all of the science-based information you need to maximize your brain health. "Science based" is key here. Social media and other online sources are full of misinformation about many topics, including aging and brain health. Even some published books exaggerate or otherwise misrepresent the state of the science. You can expect myth-busting to be a regular feature in this book.

There are quite a few myths about aging. Take the 2020 U.S. presidential election. In the months and weeks leading up to the election, how often did you hear or read disparaging comments about the age of some of the candidates? You might even have your own concerns about the ability of someone in their 70s to run the country. Jokes and memes, as well as serious commentary on this topic, have been frequent. Take, for example, a *Washington Post* op-ed piece entitled, "Joe Biden and Bernie Sanders Are Too Old to Be President" (Cohen, 2019). A few weeks later, the *Post* published an article reflecting a different perspective, entitled "No One Is Too Old to Be President" (Chappel & Edelstein, 2019). As the article's subhead aptly stated, "The Jokes and Jabs About Older Candidates Are Rooted in Ageism, Not Science."

At the heart of the disparaging comments about the age of the presidential candidates was the myth that aging inevitably signals dementia. Society often assumes that older adults are uniformly declining in capacity. This belief reflects two common misconceptions: first, that older adults are all alike and, second, that later life is marked by cognitive impairment. In reality, there are great differences among older adults in regard to health, cognitive abilities, overall functioning, and many other aspects of life. Research has shown that variability in certain characteristics among older adults can be even greater than variability among young people (e.g., Lowsky et al., 2014). And for most seniors, changes in cognitive functioning associated with aging are generally mild and do not interfere with their day-to-day life. The American Psychological Association offers a great summary of facts and myths surrounding the health of older adults on its website (https://www.apa.org/pi/aging/resources/guides/myth-reality.pdf).

Science tells us that aging is influenced both by biology (including genetics, medical conditions, and substance use) and environment. Our environment includes some things we can't change, such as our early lives and past experiences but, more important, environment also includes lifestyle, and we can make choices to have healthier lifestyles that lead to better functioning brains.

How can you sift through all of the information you're surrounded by to figure out what is backed by science and what isn't? This can be tricky, but here are a few tips:

- When looking online, rely as much as possible on information from large, reputable hospitals and other health organizations.

Examples include the National Institutes of Health, American Psychological Association, American Heart Association, Centers for Disease Control and Prevention, Mayo Clinic, and Cleveland Clinic.

- **Check the credentials of the author or speaker presenting the information.** It's important to not only look at the letters behind their name, such as PhD or MD, but to also consider their field of study and professional experience. For example, someone can have a PhD in chemistry and a successful career working for a large chemical manufacturer. These are great credentials, but they have nothing to do with brain health. Be cautious about relying on information on topics such as brain health if the information comes from an expert in an unrelated field.

- **Beware of potential traps from viral media.** Decades of research have identified what psychologists call the *illusory truth effect*. The basic idea is that we lend credibility to ideas we hear repeatedly. In a world where a sensational story or shocking information (or misinformation) so quickly goes viral, bombarding us across multiple media platforms, you can imagine how easy it is for any of us to succumb to this phenomenon. Make sure you apply the first two tips before believing supposed "facts" that are trending online!

- **Double-check your information.** As a scientist, my default is to look for verification of any information I hear. If I hear it from only one source, I take it with a grain of salt. If multiple *reputable* sources (or in the case of science, multiple research studies) point in the same direction, then my confidence in that information grows.

This book is a trustworthy, science-based source of information about brain health. I based it on more than 20 years of experience in the field of neuropsychology, as I studied the relationships between the brain and behavior and provided clinical care to clients with brain disorders. My primary source of information for this book is the vast amount of research that links certain behaviors to healthy brains, and I make a point to be clear when the body of research in a particular area is limited or not entirely consistent.

## A FEW NOTES ON SCIENCE

As you read this book, it is important to keep in mind what science is and is not. Scientific research is a systematic way of testing *hypotheses*, or tentative, proposed explanations, about our world. It is a great way of gaining knowledge because it is designed to be systematic, objective, and replicable. *Replicable* means that someone else can perform the same experiment, or one very similar to it, and get the same results. Because research studies generally involve analyzing data from dozens to thousands of participants, the information we glean is less biased than information from personal anecdotes about one or two people.

The caveat to keep in mind is that because human beings are so complex, it can be difficult to have complete consistency across studies that test the same hypotheses. Take the case of memory and depression. Many researchers, including myself, have performed studies that revealed a relationship between depressed mood and problems with memory. However, there are other researchers whose studies did not show this relationship.

There are many possible reasons for this inconsistency. Maybe the participants were more severely depressed in the studies that found a relationship, and participants had milder symptoms in those that did not find a relationship. Perhaps the different studies used different memory tests, and some tests are better at picking up on memory problems than others. Or maybe the participants were older in the studies that found a link compared with those that did not.

What this means is that it is premature to fully put your faith in just one or two research studies, because chances are there are other studies that contradict them. Instead, it is best to look for a consensus. What do the majority of studies find? There is actually a way for scientists to examine consistency using statistics. It is called a *meta-analysis*. A meta-analysis uses statistics to combine the results of many different studies into one mega-study. By doing this, a researcher is able to illuminate the overall trend of dozens or even hundreds of separate studies. I often refer to meta-analyses in this book because they can provide the most compelling evidence for the links between certain behaviors and healthy brains.

Brain health research typically falls into one of three categories: (a) cross-sectional, (b) longitudinal, and (c) intervention. To illustrate the differences, let's say I want to design a study to test the hypothesis that physical fitness is related to memory.

A *cross-sectional study* examines people at one point in time. For my physical fitness and memory idea, I might recruit 100 volunteers and have each of them come into my lab. I can ask them to learn a list of words and then test their memory for the words half an hour later. I can then give them an aerobic fitness assessment, such as a VO2 max test, which measures the body's capacity to use oxygen during exercise. Think of horsepower for your car, but for VO2 max the body is equivalent to the engine and oxygen is equivalent to fuel. With their memory test scores and VO2 max data in hand, I can perform statistical analyses to see if the people with better aerobic fitness performed better on the memory test.

If instead I planned a *longitudinal study*, the design would look a little different. Longitudinal studies test people at two or more points to assess *changes* that occur over time. In this case, I might start off giving 100 volunteers the same memory test and VO2 max test that I described for the cross-sectional study, but then I would also have the volunteers come back at a later time for more testing.

I could repeat the same tests, for example, at the first visit (this is called the *baseline* visit) and then again 6 months later. Then I could use statistics to verify whether the people who had the highest aerobic fitness at the baseline visit had better memory abilities 6 months later. This kind of question could be especially important in people with medical conditions that normally cause declines in memory, such as Alzheimer's disease.

An *intervention study* is a special type of longitudinal study. Instead of simply testing people at more than one time, the researcher systematically gives the volunteers some type of medical or psychological treatment between the baseline visit and the follow-up visit. For example, I could give 100 people the word list memory test during an initial visit to my lab. Then I would randomly put half of them in a group that comes into the lab for running sessions three times a week for 6 months. The other 50 people come into the lab three times a week for stretching sessions. Then I could test everyone's memory again after 6 months of either running or stretching. At that point, I could use statistics to see if my intervention (aerobic exercise) led to greater memory improvements after 6 months compared with the stretching sessions.

Cross-sectional, longitudinal, and intervention studies all have their pros and cons, but ultimately they provide valuable information to help us understand links between behavior and brain health. However, intervention studies give us the most confidence that certain behaviors actually cause some type of change. In the example I've been using, I would have more confidence that aerobic exercise leads to memory improvement in the intervention study because I compared changes over time in people who did and did not do the exercise. Longitudinal studies that do not involve some type of intervention still provide stronger evidence than cross-sectional studies because they test people over time to measure changes. Cross-sectional studies cannot speak to change, but they do point to possible differences. For example, my hypothetical study could show that aerobically fit people perform better on memory tests, even though I can't say for sure that it's the aerobic fitness that caused the better memory.

As you read this book and consume information about brain health from other sources, think about what you have learned about how science works, and put the most weight on the knowledge you garner from reputable sources. Now that you know what a healthy brain is and have some tips on how to keep your brain healthy, let's begin our journey!

## SUMMARY

As you read the rest of this book, remember the background information you learned in this chapter:

- Your brain is essential to every aspect of your life. A healthy brain has the blood flow it needs to power your every thought and action. This requires you to have an intact brain structure, such as the size of your brain, and healthy brain functioning of the inner workings of your brain.
- An unhealthy brain can cause a variety of problems. For example, it can affect your mood, interfere with your memory, and increase your risk for Alzheimer's disease and other types of dementia.
- Healthy behavior can benefit your brain, making it possible for you to prevent, delay, or slow down some brain diseases. There is no quick fix; achieving and keeping a healthy brain takes work and a long-term commitment. But it's never too late to start. Regardless of your age or health status, the time to focus on your brain health is now.

- The brain-healthy behaviors with the most scientific evidence include staying physically, mentally, and socially active; keeping a healthy diet and good sleep habits; and treating physical and mental health conditions.
- A healthy lifestyle can lower our risk for the ill effects of an unhealthy brain, but it cannot fully eliminate the risk. If you or a loved one has concerns about memory loss or cognitive decline, see your doctor and ask for a referral to a neuropsychologist.
- Make sure to get your information about health, including brain health, from reputable experts, not from viral media. Double-check your information instead of trusting one source.
- Scientific research is a systematic, objective way of testing hypotheses about our world. It's a great way of gaining knowledge, but it still has limitations. Because no study is perfect, different studies can contradict each other. Before you take to heart information you hear, look for consensus across multiple research studies.

## RESOURCES AND SUGGESTED READINGS

**AARP/Global Council on Brain Health:** https://www.aarp.org/health/brain-health/global-council-on-brain-health/resource-library/

This resource library provides information about various topics related to brain health. It was put together by a team of scientists, doctors, scholars, and policy experts from around the world.

**Sense about Science, "I Don't Know What to Believe" booklet:** https://senseaboutscience.org/activities/i-dont-know-what-to-believe/

This excellent eight-page booklet offers tips on how to make sense of scientific stories.

National Institute on Aging, "Cognitive Health and Older Adults": https://www.nia.nih.gov/health/cognitive-health-and-older-adults
This site provides comprehensive information about cognitive aging from one of the National Institutes of Health, including helpful tips about what is normal memory decline and what is not.

National Institute on Aging, "Memory, Forgetfulness, and Aging: What's Normal and What's Not?" https://www.nia.nih.gov/health/memory-forgetfulness-and-aging-whats-normal-and-whats-not
Information from the National Institute on Aging to help you decide when you or your loved one should see someone about memory problems.

National Institute on Aging, Caregiving Resources: https://www.nia.nih.gov/health/caregiving
A collection of resources for caregivers of people with dementia or other serious health conditions.

Alzheimer's Association, Brain Health: https://www.alz.org/help-support/brain_health
A collection of resources to learn more about healthy behaviors that promote a healthy brain.

American Heart Association, Brain Health Resources: https://www.heart.org/en/health-topics/brain-health/brain-health-resources
Another good collection of resources to learn more about healthy behaviors that promote a healthy brain.

Budson, A. E., & O'Connor, M. K. (2017). *Seven steps to managing your memory: What's normal, what's not, and what to do about it*. Oxford University Press.
This reader-friendly book addresses memory problems, including what's normal and what's not, when to see a doctor, and what resources you can use when you experience memory problems.

Wenk, G. L. (2017). *The brain: What everyone needs to know.* Oxford University Press.

This is an easy-to-read introduction to the brain, presented in a question-and-answer format that explains why it is important to everyday life.

## SELECTED REFERENCES

Arvanitakis, Z., Shah, R. C., & Bennett, D. A. (2019). Diagnosis and management of dementia: Review. *Journal of the American Medical Association, 322*(16), 1589–1599. https://doi.org/10.1001/jama.2019.4782

Chappel, J., & Edelstein, S. (2019, April 25). No one is too old to be President. *The Washington Post.* https://www.washingtonpost.com/outlook/2019/04/25/no-one-is-too-old-be-president/

Cohen, R. (2019, March 18). Joe Biden and Bernie Sanders are too old to be President. *The Washington Post.* https://www.washingtonpost.com/opinions/joe-biden-and-bernie-sanders-are-too-old-to-be-president/2019/03/18/66f9a316-49ac-11e9-93d0-64dbcf38ba41_story.html

Devitt, M. (2018). *CDC data show U.S. life expectancy continues to decline.* https://www.aafp.org/news/health-of-the-public/20181210lifeexpectdrop.html#:~:text=in%20three%20years.-,Three%20new%20reports%20from%20the%20CDC%20indicate%20that%20the%20average,to%2078.6%20years%20in%202017

Donders, J. (2020). The incremental value of neuropsychological assessment: A critical review. *The Clinical Neuropsychologist, 34*(1), 56–87. https://doi.org/10.1080/13854046.2019.1575471

Dotson, V. M. (2017). Variability in depression: What have we been missing? *American Journal of Geriatric Psychiatry, 25*(1), 23–24. https://doi.org/10.1016/j.jagp.2016.10.005

Dotson, V. M., Szymkowicz, S. M., Kim, J. U., & McClintock, S. M. (2018). Cognitive functioning in late-life depression: A critical review of sociodemographic, neurobiological, and treatment correlates. *Current Behavioral Neuroscience Reports, 5*(4), 310–318. https://doi.org/10.1007/s40473-018-0159-4

Dotson, V. M., Taiwo, Z., Minto, L. R., Bogoian, H. R., & Gradone, A. M. (2021). Orbitofrontal and cingulate thickness asymmetry associated with depressive symptom dimensions. *Cognitive, Affective, and Behavioral Neuroscience.* Advance online publication. https://doi.org/10.3758/s13415-021-00923-8

Health or finances? Older Americans and professionals who support them disagree on needs of growing aging population. (2015, July 8). https://www.n4a.org/files/USA15-National-News-Release-Final.pdf

Livingston, G., Huntley, J., Sommerlad, A., Ames, D., Ballard, C., Banerjee, S., Brayne, C., Burns, A., Cohen-Mansfield, J., Cooper, C., Costafreda, S. G., Dias, A., Fox, N., Gitlin, L. N., Howard, R., Kales, H. C., Kivimäki, M., Larson, E. B., Ogunniyi, A., . . . Mukadam, N. (2020). Dementia prevention, intervention, and care: 2020 report of the Lancet Commission. *The Lancet, 396*(10248), 413–446. https://doi.org/10.1016/S0140-6736(20)30367-6

Lowsky, D. J., Olshansky, S. J., Bhattacharya, J., & Goldman, D. P. (2014). Heterogeneity in healthy aging. *Journals of Gerontology: Series A. Biological Sciences and Medical Sciences, 69*(6), 640–649. https://doi.org/10.1093/gerona/glt162

McLaren, M. E., Szymkowicz, S. M., O'Shea, A., Woods, A. J., Anton, S. D., & Dotson, V. M. (2017). Vertex-wise examination of symptom dimensions of subthreshold depression and brain volumes. *Psychiatric Research: Neuroimaging, 260,* 70–75. https://doi.org/10.1016/j.pscychresns.2016.12.008

Michalak, H. R., King, T. Z., Turner, J. A., Semmel, E. S., & Dotson, V. M. (2020). Linking depressive symptom dimensions to cerebellar subregion volumes in later life. *Translational Psychiatry.* Advance online publication. https://doi.org/10.1038/s41398-020-00883-6

Nyberg, L., Boraxbekk, C.-J., Sörman, D. E., Hansson, P., Herlitz, A., Kauppi, K., Ljungberg, J. K., Lövheim, H., Lundquist, A., Adolfsson, A. N., Oudin, A., Pudas, S., Rönnlund, M., Stiernstedt, M., Sundström, A., & Adolfsson, R. (2020). Biological and environmental predictors of heterogeneity in neurocognitive ageing: Evidence from Betula and other longitudinal studies. *Ageing Research Reviews, 64,* 101184. https://doi.org/10.1016/j.arr.2020.101184

Randolph, J. (2020, May 6). 7 ways to promote brain health during a pandemic. *Psychology Today.* https://www.psychologytoday.com/us/blog/the-healthy-engaged-brain/202005/7-ways-promote-brain-health-during-pandemic

Santoni, G., Angleman, S., Welmer, A. K., Mangialasche, F., Marengoni, A., & Fratiglioni, L. (2015). Age-related variation in health status after age 60. *PLOS ONE, 10*(3), e0120077. https://doi.org/10.1371/journal.pone.0120077

Skufca, L. (2015, October). *2015 Survey on Brain Health.* AARP Research. https://doi.org/10.26419/res.00114.001

Szymkowicz, S. M., McLaren, M. E., Kirton, J. W., O'Shea, A., Woods, A. J., Manini, T. M., Anton, S. D., & Dotson, V. M. (2016). Depressive symptom severity is associated with increased cortical thickness in older adults. *International Journal of Geriatric Psychiatry, 31*(4), 325–333. https://doi.org/10.1002/gps.4324

# CHAPTER 2

# GET UP AND MOVE: PHYSICAL ACTIVITY FOR A HEALTHY BRAIN

She didn't always keep up with the moves, but what I noticed most about the woman in my Zumba class was the huge smile that never left her face. As she lost herself in the music, she did not seem to care that she was clearly two or three times the age of the other students, most of whom were in their 20s and 30s. I was the instructor. She came up to me afterward and said, "I just love this class! It keeps me moving and it keeps the wheels turning in my head!" Guessing that she was in her 70s, I told her that classes like Zumba are great because you can enjoy them at any age. I was thrilled when she responded, "I'm 89 years old, so if I can do it, anyone can do it!"

Little did my octogenarian student know that scientific studies back up what she said. Exercise does "keep the wheels turning!" When we think about exercising, most of us think about benefits such as a healthy heart, stronger muscles, and increased flexibility. Did you know that physical activity is also good for your brain?

In this chapter, you will learn about the many ways physical activity can lead to a healthier brain, boost your cognitive functioning, and reduce your risk of dementia. We will go over expert recommendations for what type and how much exercise is best and discuss practical suggestions for how to develop a more physically active lifestyle.

## WHAT RESEARCH TELLS US

Researchers in different fields, such as psychology, neuroscience, and exercise science study the effects of physical activity on the brain. "Physical activity" means any movement that requires energy and uses muscles. This includes activities at work or around the house that involve movement. The word "exercise" refers to structured physical activities meant to improve physical fitness. We consider activities such as running, swimming, or yoga forms of exercise because they are structured and they help to improve or maintain strength, balance, or aerobic capacity. But exercise, and even everyday physical activities, are also great ways to keep your brain healthy.

### Exercise Can Cause Certain Parts of Your Brain to Increase in Size

About 10 years ago, I had an experience that changed my career. In my first semester as a professor, I listened to one of my students give a presentation about some of the research he was doing as an undergraduate research assistant. After all of my training, I assumed I would be at least a little familiar with the topic of his presentation. But I was wrong! I learned something I had never heard before: Exercise can actually cause certain parts of your brain to increase in size. He talked about two studies that caught my attention. In one, the researchers scanned the brains of men and women between ages 55 and 79. The researchers also measured aerobic fitness. They found that some parts of the brains of the older participants were smaller than the same parts in the younger participants. This was not new: Scientists have known for years that brain size decreases as we age. What was exciting was that the people in the study who were more physically fit showed less reduction in brain size.

The second study was an intervention study. The researchers randomly separated people between ages 60 and 79 into an aerobic exercise group or a control group for 6 months. The aerobic group did exercises that increased their heart rates three times a week. The control group did stretching and toning exercises on the same schedule. At the end of the study, some parts of the brains of the people who spent 6 months doing aerobic exercises increased in size. In fact, some of these areas were the ones that tend to get smaller as we age and are linked to conditions such as Alzheimer's disease and depression.

Over the past decade, study after study has validated the ideas that captivated my attention during my student's research presentation. These studies show that people who are more active or more physically fit have larger volumes in parts of the brain, such as the frontal lobes and hippocampus, which are important for memory; attention; and what are known as *executive functions, or complex mental activities such as multitasking*. For example, one study found that people who had an exercise regimen of taking brisk walks three times a week for 1 year saw their hippocampus—an area of the brain important for memory—increase in size. In the same study, people who only performed stretching and toning exercises for the same time period saw a slight decline in the size of the hippocampus. Many researchers have also repeated the finding that people who are more fit have less age-related loss in brain tissue. In fact, older adults who have been active or fit in the past have larger brains than their inactive counterparts years after they stop exercising!

### Exercise Can Help Your Brain Function Better

At the same time, in the brain, size is not all that matters. Your brain needs to *function* well, which means that your brain cells fire when needed and that they communicate efficiently with each other.

It turns out that exercise also improves brain function. Joe Nocera is a researcher at Emory University who studies the benefits of exercise for brain function. In some of his studies, he looks at what is called the "resting state" of the brain. Resting-state studies measure blood flow in the brain while people are doing nothing but lying still inside a brain scanner. It's considered "resting" because the person is not being asked to do any kind of cognitive or motor task, unlike in a lot of other brain studies. These studies allow researchers to measure how well brain cells communicate with each other. As Nocera explains it, "The resting state is an important aspect of brain health because connectivity, or how different parts of the brain communicate with one another during the resting state, is a fundamental aspect of brain function."

In one of his recent studies, Nocera led exercise groups for older adults three times a week. Half of the participants took a spin cycling class designed to really get the heart pumping. This was aerobic exercise. The other half did a series of stretching and toning exercises in their classes. The study continued for 12 weeks. Brain scans at the end of the study showed that people who took the spin cycling classes had better communication—better connectivity—between areas of the brain that are important for motor control. Moreover, these changes were related to better performance on tasks that required motor skills, such as tapping one's finger quickly or having enough dexterity to fit small objects of different shapes into small holes in a board. When I asked Nocera what he found most exciting about his study results, he said it was the fact that older adults who had fairly inactive lifestyles before the study could see benefits after only 12 weeks of exercise. His conclusion: "It is never too late to start an exercise program and benefit from it!"

This is not the only study to show that exercise is a great way to help your brain function better. Scientists have shown that the brains of people who are more physically active function more efficiently during memory and other mental tasks. The people in research studies who have the most changes in aerobic fitness after starting an exercise program also have the most changes in brain function, and the areas of the brain that benefit the most are important for abilities such as attention.

## Exercise Can Improve the Vascular Health of Your Brain

Baby boomers—the 76 million people born between 1946 and 1964—cite heart disease as one of their biggest health concerns. You have likely heard all about a "heart-healthy" lifestyle—practices, such as eating right and exercising to control high blood pressure and high cholesterol, conditions that can lead to heart disease. A heart-healthy lifestyle is also a brain-healthy lifestyle. That is because the heart and the brain both need healthy blood vessels to supply them with oxygen and nutrients. Vascular, or blood, diseases affect the body's network of blood vessels, so they can affect the heart, the brain, or both. Conditions that affect the blood supply to the brain are called *cerebrovascular diseases*. Strokes and aneurysms are common examples. We often think about the benefits of exercise for your heart (cardiovascular health), but exercise is also important for cerebrovascular health.

I see a lot of clients who have some type of risk factor for vascular disease, such as Type 2 diabetes or high blood pressure. Most of them know that exercise is really important for their heart health, but let's face it, getting started in a regular exercise program is tough! I have found that my clients get an extra boost of motivation to exercise when they learn about the link between heart health and brain health. Regular physical activity indirectly affects brain health by reducing the risk for chronic diseases such as Type 2 diabetes and high blood pressure and by keeping these types of conditions under control in people who already have them. Aerobic exercises, such as brisk walking, running, and riding a bicycle, are especially effective ways to improve both your cardiovascular health and your cerebrovascular health.

## Exercise Can Help the Brain "Rewire"

Decades ago, scientists believed that we have a fixed number of nerve cells in the brain, so the nerve cells cannot be replaced if they are damaged or die. We now know that the brain can rewire throughout life, regardless of your age! And exercise is a great way to help rewire your brain. The term "neuroplasticity" refers to the brain's ability to reorganize itself, for example, as you learn new information or recover from brain injury or disease. Exercise promotes neuroplasticity. People who regularly exercise can increase the amount of chemicals in the brain that are important for neuroplasticity and for the overall health of brain cells. Through these chemicals, physical exercise affects the shape and size of brain cells and can even help new brain cells and blood vessels grow and develop.

## Exercise Can Improve Your Mental Abilities and Reduce Your Risk of Dementia

In my clinical practice, I most often evaluate adults over age 65 who have concerns about their cognitive abilities. What is their most common concern? Memory! Almost every client I see says things such as, "I keep misplacing my keys" or "My family complains that I don't remember conversations we had" or "I used to be good at names, but now I forget them almost as soon as I hear them." We can expect to become a bit more forgetful as we get older—it is a normal part of the aging process. Still, no one wants to have memory lapses and, even more, we don't want the memory problems to keep getting worse and develop into a serious condition such as Alzheimer's disease. I have good news for you: Exercise can improve your memory and other cognitive abilities. Furthermore, exercise can even lower your risk of developing Alzheimer's disease!

In one study, adults between ages 55 and 80 were randomly put in either a walking group or a stretching-and-toning group.

Everyone in the study exercised three times each week. Participants in the walking group started off walking 10 minutes at a time and then increased 5 minutes each week until they reached 40-minute sessions. The stretching-and-toning group was used as a control group because stretching is not considered an aerobic exercise and the researchers wanted to learn more about how aerobic exercise affects memory. Stretching-and-toning sessions involved a combination of muscle-building exercises and balance exercises. Everyone in the study received brain scans before starting their exercise program, 6 months into the study, and again after they had been in the study for 1 year. At those same time points, they completed a computerized memory test that required them to remember the location of dots that had flashed on the screen. The researchers found that, for people in the aerobic exercise group, the size of a portion of the hippocampus increased over the course of the study. They also found that the more the hippocampus grew, the better the person's memory was at the end of the study.

This connection between exercise and memory makes sense. A healthy brain is important for cognitive abilities such as memory. Because exercise can lead to a healthier brain, it is not surprising that research studies have shown that exercise also benefits memory and other cognitive abilities. Many studies suggest that people who are more physically fit not only have a better memory but also score better on tests measuring attention and mental speed. One study followed people for up to 10 years and found that physically active older adults had less decline over time in their cognitive skills compared with their less active peers. Other studies have shown that older adults who exercise regularly and increase their physical fitness often improve these skills.

Many different types of cognitive abilities can improve after regular aerobic exercise, but *executive functions*—different skills that we use to control and coordinate our other cognitive abilities and behaviors—improve the most. Think of an executive of a company as the person who runs the show, ensuring that employees work together to meet the company's goals. Some of the cognitive skills that scientists refer to as executive functions are things such as managing time, switching focus, planning and organizing, inhibiting ourselves by avoiding saying or doing something at the wrong time, and multitasking.

Executive functions are very important for functioning well in our everyday lives. People who have difficulty with these skills often have trouble with activities such as driving, cooking, managing medications and appointments, and other daily tasks that we must perform to live independently. Knowing that exercise can improve these skills is a great motivation to get moving.

What about people who develop very severe problems with their memory and other cognitive skills as they get older? People who report being physically active in their 40s and later in life have a lower risk of developing *mild cognitive impairment*, or cognitive decline that is more severe than expected as we grow older but not severe enough to be considered dementia. If you haven't kept a physically active lifestyle earlier in life, you can still reduce your risk if you get moving now! Research also tells us older adults who start a structured exercise program are less likely to develop mild cognitive impairment and different types of dementia, including Alzheimer's disease. This makes sense because a few studies suggest that you can reduce the growth of unhealthy brain tissue linked to Alzheimer's by keeping a physically active lifestyle. Older adults who exercised three or more times a week had as much as a 32% reduction in their risk for developing dementia during a 6-year period, according to researchers from a longitudinal study called the Adult Changes in Thought Study.

In people who already have Alzheimer's disease, a higher level of physical fitness is linked to larger brain volume, especially in the hippocampus, a brain region that is strongly linked to Alzheimer's.

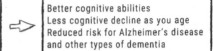

## YOUR BRAIN ON EXERCISE

| | |
|---|---|
| Some areas of the brain get bigger. The brain functions more efficiently. The brain is better able to repair itself and grow new cells. Blood supply in the brain gets better. | Better cognitive abilities Less cognitive decline as you age Reduced risk for Alzheimer's disease and other types of dementia |

Research shows that people with other types of dementia, such as dementia caused by damage to the brain's vascular system, can also get a brain boost if they exercise regularly. People with dementia who participate in a physical activity involving aerobic exercise, or even a slower exercise, such as tai chi, are able to slow down their memory decline. Because there is no cure for dementia, physical activity is a really important strategy to prevent the disease—or, if you have the disease, to live a better, more rewarding life.

### What Kind of Exercise, and How Often?

When I give presentations about exercise and brain health to the community or to other psychologists, I constantly hear two questions: What is the best type of exercise? How much exercise is enough? The simple answer is this: Any physical activity is better than no physical activity! But what else does research tell us about these two important questions?

When it comes to the best type of exercise, the good news is, research shows that a wide variety of exercises can help you achieve a healthy brain. However, aerobic exercise seems to give you the most bang for your buck. Remember, what's good for your heart is good for your brain. The more you get your heart pumping when you exercise, the more you benefit your brain.

But even though intense aerobic activities such as running are great, many studies have shown that low-intensity aerobics can improve your brain health, too. For example, after inactive older adults participated in 6 to 12 months of a walking program, different areas of the brain important to cognitive functioning increased in size. They also saw improved vascular health in their brains after 12 months in the walking program. Recent research suggests that your best bet might be to vary your aerobic exercise intensity through interval training (e.g., 3 minutes low intensity/3 minutes high intensity) rather than keeping steady exercise at the same intensity.

But it's not only aerobic exercise that helps. Adults in their 40s, 50s, and older who regularly engage in exercises such as stretching and resistance training have better memory than people who are inactive. Some researchers recommend a combination of aerobic and resistance training to get the best results. You can also achieve a healthier brain through mind–body exercises such as yoga, Pilates, and tai chi. If you find it hard to get started with structured exercises, you still have options! You can improve your brain health by doing more of your everyday activities, such as housework or gardening.

The next question is, how much exercise is enough? Again, *any* exercise is better than none. But many researchers and health

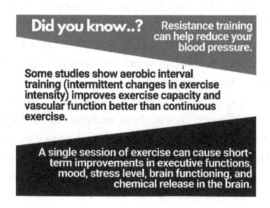

**Did you know..?** Resistance training can help reduce your blood pressure.

Some studies show aerobic interval training (intermittent changes in exercise intensity) improves exercise capacity and vascular function better than continuous exercise.

A single session of exercise can cause short-term improvements in executive functions, mood, stress level, brain functioning, and chemical release in the brain.

care providers stick to recommendations by the American Heart Association and the American College of Sports Medicine, which advise adults over the age of 18 to aim for the following:

- moderate-intensity aerobic activity for a minimum of 150 minutes each week, or
- vigorous-intensity aerobic activity for a minimum of 75 minutes each week, and
- muscle-strengthening exercises for a minimum of 2 days each week.

Moderate-intensity aerobic exercises should make you feel warm and start to break a sweat. Your breathing should be hard enough that you can talk but not sing your favorite song. Moderate-intensity exercises include brisk walking, using a stair climber or elliptical, water aerobics classes, or even playing actively with your children or grandchildren.

Vigorous-intensity aerobic exercises should make you feel hot and sweaty and raise your heart rate quite a bit. You should feel breathless. You should not be able to say more than a few words without taking a breath. Some examples are running, playing a sport such as soccer or basketball, and high-impact dance classes.

A good goal is to add balance, coordination, and flexibility exercises 2 days each week. Balance training is especially important as you get older. The World Health Organization recommends that people 65 and older work on what's called *functional balance* three times each week. Functional balance exercises require you to maintain a position that requires balance, such as standing on one foot, and keep that position stable even when you make another movement, such as lifting one knee while the other leg balances you. These types of exercises can help you strengthen muscles that keep your body upright, which helps prevent falls.

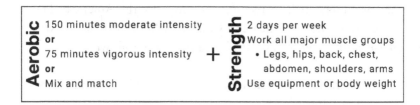

These are general guidelines. Depending on your age, sex, and risk for heart disease, your exercise goals might be different. For example, the World Health Organization (2020) offers guidelines for different age groups, from infancy to 65+. Before starting to exercise, you might talk to your doctor to see what guidelines you should follow.

You might also be wondering how quickly you can expect to see results. In some studies, people perform better on memory tests after as few as 3 months of regular exercise, but most studies show improvements in brain health, such as better memory or more efficient processing, after 6 to 12 months. With this in mind, you should plan to make regular exercise part of a *lifestyle change*, not a short-term commitment.

There is, however, a good chance for short-term benefits from exercise too. A single exercise session can have great short-term benefits! Researchers have found small improvements in cognitive performance and brain functioning after a single session of exercise. This effect might be linked to a release of chemicals in the brain that are important for your brain health. You might have noticed that sometimes you feel better emotionally after a good workout; this is sometimes called a "runner's high." Research shows the reason for this. A single session of exercise can improve your mood by increasing positive feelings, decreasing negative feelings, and reducing your level of stress. These short-term effects can last for up to 2 hours after an exercise session.

I like to use this to my advantage at work. I usually work out either first thing in the morning or around lunchtime. Exercising

| Practical Tips for Physical Activity | | | |
|---|---|---|---|
| Do more of your current physical activities, unless you're extremely active already | Try new activities you think you will enjoy | A variety of physical activities is better than one kind alone | In a safe community or area, walk to your destination |
| Take the stairs instead of the elevator | Park farther away from your destination | Engage in active hobbies such as gardening and dancing | Get moving throughout your day |
| Challenge yourself a little bit more over time | Be patient and persistent | To stay motivated, consider doing physical activities with other people | Make concrete plans to move your body |

*Note.* From "The Brain–Body Connection: GCBH Recommendations on Physical Activity and Brain Health," July 2016 (https://www.aarp.org/content/dam/aarp/health/brain_health/2016/05/gcbh-physical-activity-and-brain-health-report-english-aarp.doi.10.26419%252Fpia.00013.001.pdf). Copyright 2016 by the Global Council on Brain Health. Adapted with permission.

first thing helps me wake up—even if it is hard to get started!—and helps me focus when I get to work. I get a midafternoon boost when I exercise in the middle of the day. Instead of having an afternoon slump in energy and focus, I find that I am energized and more productive.

## LET'S GET MOVING! PLANNING FOR YOUR PHYSICALLY ACTIVE LIFE

Meet Jay. Jay is one of five people in my personal training group. Twice a week, we attend sessions with our personal trainer, who gives us a grueling mix of aerobic and resistance exercises for 45 minutes. These personal training sessions are intense! Jay has been a part of the group for 2 years. He has rarely missed a session. He brings his

A game every single day. He is able to complete challenging exercises, such as pull-ups, that other group members struggle to perform. And he is 60 years old. Because I have such a strong personal and professional interest in encouraging everyone to exercise to achieve a healthy brain, regardless of age, you can imagine how excited I am to have Jay in my personal training group. I spoke with him to find out how he keeps himself active in his sixth decade of life. Here is what I learned.

In his late 50s, Jay noticed that he was putting on the pounds, so he changed his eating habits to shed the extra weight. Once he reached his goal weight, he decided an exercise program would be a good way to maintain a healthy weight. That's when he joined our personal training group. He finds it helpful to have the structure and social aspects of the training group and to have guidance from a trainer who understands his goals and can help him reach those goals. But he didn't stop at the twice-per-week training sessions; he also finds ways to stay active throughout the week. He goes for walks three to four times each week. Sometimes this is as simple as walking instead of driving to the grocery store a quarter mile from his house. When he is running errands, he leaves his car parked in one spot and walks to other nearby stores instead of moving his car to go to each store. He has even found creative ways to stay active at work! He makes a point to get up and walk around two or three times each day. He figured out a route between buildings on his work campus that totals about 1 mile, so he intentionally walks that entire route for exercise.

Jay has seen many gains from his new active lifestyle. Not only has he stayed at his target weight and lowered his blood pressure, but he also sleeps better and is more focused at work. These benefits keep him motivated to continue his exercise regimen. It's no wonder he rarely misses a personal training session. Physical activity has become an important part of his life. He told me, "I'm miserable if I miss. I look forward to it." After seeing so many positives from regular exercise, he said, "I wish I had the desire to exercise in my 30s!"

Jay is a great example of what it takes to start and maintain a physically active lifestyle. Now that you know the science behind exercise and brain health, the next step is for you to get moving, too! Jay's story highlights a very important point about starting an exercise program: You have to *plan* for it. Make exercise a part of your week, not something that you try to squeeze in at the last minute. Schedule your exercise sessions like you would schedule a doctor's appointment or a get-together with friends or family. It's easy to get caught up in a busy schedule and push this part of your life to the side, but make it a priority to stick to your schedule unless there is an emergency or you are physically unable because of injury or illness. Make a plan that makes sense for your schedule, your age and health, and your resources. You are more likely to stick to a plan if you have a feeling of success early on.

Think about what helps you stay organized and on track in other areas of your life, and see if you can use the same strategies for starting and maintaining a physically active lifestyle. Keep a weekly calendar or exercise log to help you plan your activities in advance and track your activities over time. You might want to try one of the many websites and smartphone apps that have been developed to track physical activity. A few examples are provided at the end of this chapter.

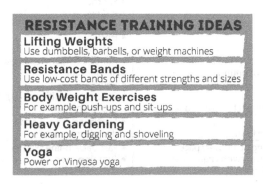

**RESISTANCE TRAINING IDEAS**

**Lifting Weights**
Use dumbbells, barbells, or weight machines

**Resistance Bands**
Use low-cost bands of different strengths and sizes

**Body Weight Exercises**
For example, push-ups and sit-ups

**Heavy Gardening**
For example, digging and shoveling

**Yoga**
Power or Vinyasa yoga

Begin by picking activities that can become part of your new active lifestyle. Remember these two overarching exercise guidelines: (a) Include both aerobic and resistance exercises in your plan and (b) Choose exercises on the basis of your capabilities. If you have balance problems, for example, you might choose chair exercises or exercise machines that can be used in a sitting position.

**IDEAS FOR MODERATE AND VIGOROUS PHYSICAL ACTIVITY**

| Moderate Intensity | Vigorous Intensity |
|---|---|
| GENERAL EXERCISE | |
| • Brisk walking (3–4.5 mph) | • Walking uphill<br>• Backpacking<br>• Race walking (more than 4.5 mph)<br>• Jogging or running |
| • Stationary bicycling (slower than 10 mph) | • Stationary bicycling (10 mph or faster) |
| • Other aerobic machines (e.g., stair climber, elliptical)—moderate pace | • Other aerobic machines (e.g., stair climber, elliptical)—vigorous pace |
| • Light to moderate calisthenics (e.g., home exercises, back exercises, getting up and down from the floor) | • Heavy calisthenics (e.g., push-ups, sit-ups, jumping jacks) |
| • Low-impact aerobic dancing (e.g., Zumba Gold)<br>• Ballroom dancing<br>• Line dancing<br>• Square dancing<br>• Folk dancing | • High impact aerobic dancing (e.g., regular Zumba) |
| • Softball—fast or slow pitch<br>• Basketball—shooting baskets<br>• Badminton<br>• Volleyball<br>• Frisbee<br>• Juggling<br>• Curling<br>• Cricket—batting and bowling<br>• Archery (nonhunting)<br>• Fencing<br>• Bowling<br>• Other low-impact sports and games | • Basketball<br>• Soccer<br>• Football<br>• Rugby<br>• Kickball<br>• Hockey<br>• Lacrosse<br>• Handball—general or team<br>• Racquetball<br>• Squash<br>• Other competitive or higher impact sports and games |
| • Yoga<br>• Tai chi (long form) | • Martial arts (e.g., karate, judo, tae kwon do, jujitsu) |
| • Roller skating at leisurely pace<br>• Playing actively with children or grandchildren | • Fast pace in-line skating<br>• Jumping rope |

## IDEAS FOR MODERATE AND VIGOROUS PHYSICAL ACTIVITY

| Moderate Intensity | Vigorous Intensity |
|---|---|
| **WATER EXERCISES** ||
| • Treading water with moderate effort | • Treading water with fast, vigorous effort |
| • Water aerobics or water calisthenics | • Swimming laps with fast, vigorous effort |
| • Kayaking, canoeing | • Water jogging |
| • Springboard or platform diving | • Rowing a canoe in competition |
| • Paddle boating | • Skin diving and scuba diving |
|  | • Water polo |
| **OUTDOOR ACTIVITIES** ||
| • Golf (carrying clubs) | • Horseback riding—trotting or galloping |
| • Fishing and hunting | • Mountain biking |
| • Ice skating at a leisurely pace (9 mph or less) | • Ice skating quickly (more than 9 mph) |
| • Tennis (doubles) | • Tennis (singles) |
| • Downhill skiing—with light effort | • Downhill skiing—racing or with vigorous effort |
| • Snowmobiling | • Snowshoeing and cross-country skiing |
| • Ice sailing | • Sledding |
|  | • Tobogganing |
|  | • Playing ice hockey |
| • Children's games, like hopscotch, 4-square, and dodgeball | |
| • Playing on playground equipment | |
| **HOUSE AND YARD WORK** ||
| • Sweeping, vacuuming, and mopping floors | • Carrying groceries upstairs |
| • Washing the dog | |
| • Washing the car with vigorous effort | • Baling hay or cleaning the barn with vigorous effort |
| • Shoveling snow | • Pushing nonmotorized lawn mower |
| • Digging in the garden | • Heavy gardening (continuous digging or hoeing) |
| • Mowing or raking the lawn | |

Keep these things in mind for your aerobic exercises:

- Aerobic activity should get you breathing harder and raise your heart rate. A good goal is to do aerobic exercises 3 to 5 days each week.
- You can do a mix of moderate and vigorous aerobic activity each week, or choose one or the other. As a rule of thumb, 1 minute of vigorous activity—such as running—is about the same as 2 minutes of moderate activity—such as jogging.

- If you don't have 30 minutes at one time to exercise, don't worry! Ten-minute bouts of aerobic exercise can improve aerobic fitness, which is what you need for a healthier brain.

Keep these things in mind for your resistance exercises:

- You need to do things to strengthen your muscles at least 2 days each week. Resistance training can be any exercise that builds strength in your muscles by using an "opposing" force. The opposing force can come from your own body, such as doing push-ups and sit-ups, or it can come from exercise equipment, such as dumbbells or resistance bands. These activities should work all the major muscle groups of your body: legs, hips, back, chest, abdomen, shoulders, and arms.
- For each muscle group, try to do at least one set of resistance exercise, but aim for two or three sets. A set is eight to 12 repetitions, or complete movement of an activity, such as lifting a dumbbell. Make sure that you challenge yourself! You should do resistance exercises to the point that it's hard for you to do another repetition without help.
- You can do resistance and aerobic activities on the same day or on different days. You might want to try alternating between bouts of aerobic and resistance activity in the same workout session.

Another thing to keep in mind is, what do you enjoy? The best way to stay motivated to exercise is to find activities that fit your personality and lifestyle. Research shows that people who enjoy their exercises are more likely to stay active 6 months later compared with people who do not enjoy what they are doing. It's also important to choose activities that you feel capable of performing so that you do not get discouraged. The Brainstorming Enjoyable Physical Activities worksheet (see Exhibit 2.1) can help you come up with ideas for

**EXHIBIT 2.1. Brainstorming Enjoyable Physical Activities**

| Physical activities I *enjoy* | Where can I do it? | Who can I do it with? |
| --- | --- | --- |
| | | |
| | | |

| Physical activities I'm *willing to try* | Where can I do it? | Who can I do it with? |
| --- | --- | --- |
| | | |
| | | |

exercises you might enjoy. Write down a few activities that you already know you enjoy—perhaps things you're already doing or used to do in the past. Also think about new physical activities that you haven't tried but sound like fun. For both new and old activities, think about the practical details, such as where you can do them and who might join you. Having a workout buddy can be a great way to stay motivated and have fun.

### Think Safety!

Safety is key to a smart start. You want to avoid serious medical complications caused by performing physical activities that are dangerous if you have particular medical conditions. For example, resistance training can create a sharp rise in blood pressure when you contract your muscles, so your doctor might have safety recommendations if you have severe uncontrolled high blood pressure. Other activities, such as riding a bicycle outside, can increase your risk for a fall if you have dizzy spells. Make sure you can safely exercise given your age, health condition, and overall lifestyle. Regardless of your age or physical limitations, you can find a way to be active and safe!

Nate Anthony is the personal trainer who leads the training group sessions that Jay and I attend, and he is the fitness manager and personal trainer for my company, CerebroFit. He is an exercise scientist, certified in functional movement screening—this means he is an expert in evaluating how you move and using that information to help you choose the best exercises for your body and to reduce the risk of injury when you exercise. In addition to personal training, he leads group fitness classes for students of all ages, including older adults. I asked him what safety recommendations he would give to someone who is getting started in a new exercise program. He offered three key pieces of advice. First, receive a physical from your doctor before getting started to make sure you don't have any physical issues that will limit you. According to health professionals, this recommendation is even more important if you

- are over the age of 65 and are not used to exercising;
- have heart trouble;
- have dizzy spells, chest pains, or shortness of breath;
- have risk factors for a heart attack and stroke, such as high blood pressure or high cholesterol;
- have been diagnosed with diabetes;
- have a history of smoking;
- are obese (a body mass index $\geq$ 30);
- have a respiratory illness, such as asthma;
- have a joint or bone disease, such as arthritis or osteoporosis;
- have a neurological illness, and/or
- experience ankle swelling (especially at night) or have lower leg pain when you walk that goes away with rest.

Nate's second recommendation is to start off slowly. As an example, he said, "Individuals who have been inactive for years should start off by walking instead of jumping right back into jogging or running." You can also gradually increase the length of your workouts. For example, if your goal is to walk 30 minutes every day, start by taking 10-minute walks 3 days a week. After a week, add a few minutes every day, or add another day to your schedule. For resistance training, Nate added, "I recommend you start off doing body weight exercises instead of jumping straight back into weights." If you're interested in group fitness classes, take beginner classes, such as restorative yoga, functional stretching, or cycling. Find out information about the intensity level of the class before you try it out, but remember that you can always go at your own pace during classes. Nate recommends that you speak to the instructor before the class to let them know that you are getting back into exercising and may need modifications for certain exercises. By starting your exercise program gradually, you can help prevent injury and limit how sore you'll feel after your workout.

The third, and biggest, safety recommendation Nate offered was, "Listen to your body. Your body will let you know when you are over-working or when you have had enough." He highlighted a few warning signs your body might give you to tell you that you should stop:

- *Elevated heart rate.* As a beginner, you'll want to stay within 60% to 70% of your maximum heart rate zone. You can get a quick estimate of your maximum heart rate using the formula "220 – age." For example, if you are 55 years old, your maximum heart rate would be 165, which is 220 – 55. This means that if you're new to exercising, your heart rate should not get higher than 99 to 116 beats per minute, which is 60% to 70% of 165.
- *Flushed or pale face.* This could be a sign that you are over-extending yourself or moving too fast. You might also have a flushed or pale face if you haven't eaten at least 2 hours before exercising, which can cause your blood sugar level to drop. If this happens, slow down and drink some water.
- *Cramping.* This means you have overworked the muscle or area of the body that is cramping. This might also be a sign that you are lacking potassium, sodium, or iron. You can prevent cramps by stretching and by drinking lots of water before and during your workout.
- *Feeling lightheaded.* Stop if you feel faint or dizzy.
- *Overheating.* Signs of overheating include headache, dizziness, nausea, faintness, cramps, or heart palpitations. Stop and drink plenty of water if this happens. Call 911 if your symptoms are severe or do not get better after you drink water and rest for a few minutes.

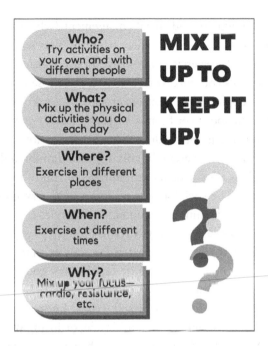

**Variety Is the Spice of Life**

As you plan your exercise program, make sure to mix it up! You already know that you should include a combination of aerobic and resistance exercises in your plan and, even better, flexibility and balance activities. You can add even more variety to keep it fresh, avoid boredom, and get the maximum health benefit. Mix up your workouts by changing the five W's:

1. *Who?* Sticking to an exercise routine is much easier—and more fun—if you have a partner. You and your partner can keep each other motivated and remind each other how far you've come! Plus, when you engage in physical activity with a partner, you are completing two parts of brain health at once:

physical activity and social engagement (which we discuss in Chapter 4). Some researchers even say that social support is necessary for exercise to improve brain health. Try a mixture of activities you can do on your own and those you can do with other people. Try a group exercise class, take walks or runs with your spouse or friends, or play outdoor games with your children and grandchildren. Even if you do not have a partner each time you exercise, involving your family and friends in your plans allows them to encourage you and check in on your progress. The social aspect of exercise is very important for building and maintaining an active lifestyle.

2. *What?* There are so many ways to be active—why stick to just one? Even if you have a particular activity that you enjoy the most—say, Zumba classes or tennis—it's good to add other activities, such as walking, jumping rope, or swimming. And you don't have to limit yourself to well-known exercise activities such as running, riding a bicycle, or lifting weights. There are many options for getting your heart rate up and strengthening your muscles! Be creative and think of ways to increase your physical activity, even for bouts of 10 minutes at a time.

3. *Where?* Mix up the route you take for walks and bike rides. Try a different room in your house for your exercises or stretching. Mix up exercising outdoors, when weather permits, and indoors. If you have access to a gym, you can use the gym some days and exercise at home or at other places in your community on other days.

4. *When?* You might want to try doing your exercises at different times and for different amounts of time. For example, try exercising in the early morning or after work if you get bored with your regular noon walk. This might not be useful for everyone. Routine can help when making lifestyle changes, so if you need to have a consistent time set aside for exercising every

day, it's better to add variety in another way instead of varying the time of day.

5. *Why?* Vary your exercise target—cardiovascular health (aerobic), strength (resistance training), flexibility and balance (yoga, tai chi, etc.), and coordination. This will not only help you meet recommended exercise guidelines but also keep things interesting because your activities will be different each day.

*Cross-training* is an exercise program that uses different activities to create a balanced fitness program. Research has shown that

☑ **Check out community organizations near you for fitness programs for older adults**

- ☐ Senior centers
- ☐ Community centers
- ☐ Recreation centers
- ☐ YMCAs, YWCAs, and local gyms
- ☐ Hospitals
- ☐ Senior living communities
- ☐ Religious groups and places of worship
- ☐ Shopping malls

**Contact your local Area Agency on Aging (https://www.n4a.org/), which might be able to help you locate senior fitness classes and transportation services.**

cross-training prevents boredom, helps you stick to your exercise plan, keeps balance among your muscle groups, and reduces your risk of injury because your muscles are not overworked by being stressed in the same way in every workout.

## Tips for Success

Starting and maintaining a physically active life takes effort. If you find ways to have fun, set realistic goals, and think of solutions to any barriers, you will be more likely to reach your goals.

### MAKE IT FUN!

Whatever activities you choose, find ways to have as much fun as possible. The best activities are the ones that you can't wait to do again, such as a spin class if you like riding bikes, or a hike if you love the outdoors. Taking a group fitness class can increase the fun element if you love being around people, plus it helps keep you accountable. Even if you're using exercise equipment or taking a walk on your own, listen to upbeat, enjoyable music that keeps you motivated, and don't be afraid to move to the beat!

### BE REALISTIC

Be realistic about your expectations of yourself. Slip-ups happen, so don't be too discouraged when you don't meet your goals for the week. Try to learn from the experience and see what you can change to reach your goals next week. Lifestyle change takes time and effort, but the rewards are worth it.

### ANTICIPATE BARRIERS AND THINK OF SOLUTIONS

Keeping an active lifestyle can be difficult, especially if you have to change your usual habits. Lots of barriers can get in the way, whether these are internal barriers, such as low motivation, or external ones, such as time constraints or financial limitations. But most of these barriers can be overcome, at least to some degree, with a little bit of creative thinking. Think about possible barriers now so that you can plan ahead for how to deal with them. You can use the Personal Exercise Barriers and Possible Solutions worksheet (Exhibit 2.2) to list your personal barriers and brainstorm solutions to help you overcome them so you can start and maintain a physically active life.

## SUMMARY

To wrap up, remember these key points:

- Research shows that being physically active can lead to a healthier brain.
- Some of the benefits of physical activity for your brain include increasing the size of certain parts of your brain that are important for memory and other cognitive abilities, healthier blood vessels in your brain, and better communication between brain cells.
- Physical activity can also minimize the decline in memory and other cognitive skills that usually happens as you get older, and it can decrease your risk for Alzheimer's disease and other types of dementia.
- Aim for including both aerobic exercises and muscle building, or resistance, exercises in your physical activity plan.
- Aerobic activities can include 150 minutes per week of moderate intensity exercises or 75 minutes per week of vigorous intensity exercises. Resistance exercises should include all major muscle groups and should be done twice each week.
- Even 10-minute bouts of activity can help you reach your weekly goal.

**EXHIBIT 2.2. Personal Exercise Barriers and Possible Solutions**

| My Barriers | Possible Solution |
|---|---|
|  |  |

## BARRIERS TO PHYSICAL ACTIVITY AND POSSIBLE SOLUTIONS

### BUSY SCHEDULE

Exercise first thing in the morning before your day gets busy. Try shorter periods of activity throughout the day, such as a few 10-minute walks. Combine physical activity with a task that's already part of your day, such as walking the dog or doing household chores. Think of ways to manage your time better. Ask your family for help with fitting in some time for exercise.

### FEELING SELF-CONSCIOUS IN GROUPS

Join a group or take a class with others who look or feel like you do. Start with walking, or try an exercise DVD at home. Work with a fitness expert for a few sessions to help you get started.

### PHYSICAL CONCERNS

Consult your doctor to see what exercises you can do safely. Have someone with experience watch you exercise to see if you are doing something that may put you at risk for injury. If your condition stops you from meeting the minimum guidelines, try to do as much as you can.

### BAD WEATHER

Try a variety of indoor and outdoor activities. When it's cold, hot, or humid, take precautions, or exercise indoors.

### LIMITED FINANCES

Walking is a great, free way to exercise! If the weather doesn't permit walking outside, try mall walking. Work physical activity into your day by parking farther away so you have a longer walk into the store, or taking the stairs instead of the elevator. Exercise with low-cost items such as a jump rope or elastic bands. Or use items you already have, such as using cans or milk jugs filled with water as weights for arm exercises. Do resistance exercises like push-ups or squats. If you have a TV or access to the internet, follow exercise videos that are available for no additional cost. Check with your local parks and recreation department or senior center about free or low-cost exercise programs in your area.

### FEAR OF FAILURE

Carefully define "success" and "failure" using realistic goals. If your goal is simply to become more active than you are now, it will be hard to fail. If your goal is to look like the people in health club ads or to lose a certain amount of weight, then the fear of failure is likely to hold you back.

### BALANCE OR MOBILITY PROBLEMS

Try seated exercises. You can get a full-body workout in your chair! You can also try activities such as seated volleyball and wheelchair basketball. If you have balance problems, use a recumbent stationary bicycle.

### LACK OF TRANSPORTATION

Choose an exercise partner who has reliable transportation. Use public transportation, if available. Many communities offer transportation services for individuals who are unable to drive, such as volunteer driver programs, transportation voucher programs, and escort services. Go to https://eldercare.acl.gov/ to find transportation services in your local community.

- To stay motivated, pick activities that you enjoy, keep variety in your activities, and, when possible, include a partner or exercise group.
- Consult your doctor or an exercise specialist before starting an exercise program if you have any major health concerns or have not been physically active before now.
- Plan for your physical activities the same way you would any other important appointment or weekly activity: Make it a priority, and think of ways to overcome obstacles that arise.
- Make it fun! You'll stick to a physically active lifestyle if the activities do not feel like a chore. Be creative and find ways to make your exercise plan feel less like work and more like something to enjoy.

## RESOURCES AND SUGGESTED READINGS

**Global Council on Brain Health, "The Brain–Body Connection":** https://www.aarp.org/content/dam/aarp/health/brain_health/2016/05/gcbh-physical-activity-and-brain-health-report-english-aarp.doi.10.26419%252Fpia.00013.001.pdf
Science-based recommendations for boosting brain health through physical activity from an international group of brain experts.

**Canadian Society for Exercise Physiology, "Get Active Questionnaire":** https://csep.ca/2021/01/20/pre-screening-for-physical-activity/
Brief questionnaire you can take to find out if you should seek advice from your doctor or a qualified exercise professional before becoming more physically active.

**World Health Organization Guidelines on Physical Activity and Sedentary Behavior:** https://www.who.int/news-room/fact-sheets/detail/physical-activity

Physical activity recommendations for different age groups (from infancy to 65+) and for people living with chronic illness or disability.

**National Institute on Aging, Exercise and Physical Activity:** https://www.nia.nih.gov/health/exercise-physical-activity

Comprehensive website that provides resources to help you fit exercise and physical activity into your daily life, including exercise suggestions, educational material, tip sheets, and downloadable exercise plans and progress trackers. Suggested pages on this site include:

- Exercise and Physical Activity Tracking Tools: https://www.nia.nih.gov/health/exercise-and-physical-activity-tracking-tools
- Participating in Activities You Enjoy: https://www.nia.nih.gov/health/participating-activities-you-enjoy

**Harvard Medical School, "Healthy Aging":** https://www.health.harvard.edu/aging/starting-to-exercise

Link to a short book that answers questions about physical activity and guides you through starting and maintaining an exercise program. You can purchase a print copy or an e-book from this website.

**National Center on Health, Physical Activity, and Disability:** http://www.nchpad.org/

Resource center on health promotion for people with disability.

**National Council on Aging, "Exercise & Fitness for Older Adults":** https://www.ncoa.org/older-adults/health/exercise-fitness

This site contains a list of community physical activity programs for older adults that are supported by scientific evidence. Find out more information about the program and check to see if one is available in your area.

Centers for Disease Control and Prevention, "My Physical Activity Tracker": https://www.cdc.gov/nccdphp/dnpa/physical/pdf/my_physical_activity_tracker.pdf
Link to a physical activity log in pdf format.

## SELECTED REFERENCES

Basso, J. C., & Suzuki, W. A. (2017). The effects of acute exercise on mood, cognition, neurophysiology, and neurochemical pathways: A review. *Brain Plasticity*, 2(2), 127–152. https://doi.org/10.3233/BPL-160040

Colcombe, S. J., Erickson, K. I., Raz, N., Webb, A. G., Cohen, N. J., McAuley, E., & Kramer, A. F. (2003). Aerobic fitness reduces brain tissue loss in aging humans. *Journals of Gerontology: Series A. Biological Sciences and Medical Sciences*, 58(2), 176–180. https://doi.org/10.1093/gerona/58.2.m176

Colcombe, S. J., Erickson, K. I., Scalf, P. E., Kim, J. S., Prakash, R., McAuley, E., Elavsky, S., Marquez, D. X., Hu, L., & Kramer, A. F. (2006). Aerobic exercise training increases brain volume in aging humans. *Journals of Gerontology: Series A. Biological Sciences and Medical Sciences*, 61(11), 1166–1170. https://doi.org/10.1093/gerona/61.11.1166

Erickson, K. I., Voss, M. W., Prakash, R. S., Basak, C., Szabo, A., Chaddock, L., Kim, J. S., Heo, S., Alves, H., White, S. M., Wojcicki, T. R., Mailey, E., Vieira, V. J., Martin, S. A., Pence, B. D., Woods, J. A., McAuley, E., & Kramer, A. F. (2011). Exercise training increases size of hippocampus and improves memory. *Proceedings of the National Academy of Sciences*, 108(7), 3017–3022. https://doi.org/10.1073/pnas.1015950108

Hamer, M., Muniz Terrera, G., & Demakakos, P. (2018). Physical activity and trajectories in cognitive function: English Longitudinal Study of Ageing. *Journal of Epidemiology and Community Health*, 72(6), 477–483. https://doi.org/10.1136/jech-2017-210228

Koblinsky, N. D., Meusel, L. C., Greenwood, C. E., & Anderson, N. D. (2021). Household physical activity is positively associated with gray matter volume in older adults. *BMC Geriatrics*, 21(1), 104. https://doi.org/10.1186/s12877-021-02054-8

Larson, E. B., Wang, L., Bowen, J. D., McCormick, W. C., Teri, L., Crane, P., & Kukull, W. (2006). Exercise is associated with reduced risk for incident dementia among persons 65 years of age and older. *Annals of Internal Medicine, 144*(2), 73–81. https://doi.org/10.7326/0003-4819-144-2-200601170-00004

Law, C. K., Lam, F. M., Chung, R. C., & Pang, M. Y. (2020). Physical exercise attenuates cognitive decline and reduces behavioural problems in people with mild cognitive impairment and dementia: A systematic review. *Journal of Physiotherapy, 66*(1), 9–18. https://doi.org/10.1016/j.jphys.2019.11.014

Marinus, N., Hansen, D., Feys, P., Meesen, R., Timmermans, A., & Spildooren, J. (2019). The impact of different types of exercise training on peripheral blood brain-derived neurotrophic factor concentrations in older adults: A meta-analysis. *Sports Medicine, 49*(10), 1529–1546. https://doi.org/10.1007/s40279-019-01148-z

Martland, R., Mondelli, V., Gaughran, F. & Stubbs, B. (2020). Can high-intensity interval training improve physical and mental health outcomes? A meta-review of 33 systematic reviews across the lifespan. *Journal of Sports Sciences, 38*(4), 430–469. https://doi.org/10.1080/02640414.2019.1706829

McGregor, K. M., Crosson, B., Krishnamurthy, L. C., Krishnamurthy, V., Hortman, K., Gopinath, K., Mammino, K. M., Omar, J., & Nocera, J. R. (2018). Effects of a 12-week aerobic spin intervention on resting state networks in previously sedentary older adults. *Frontiers in Psychology, 9*, 2376. https://doi.org/10.3389/fpsyg.2018.02376

Quigley, A., MacKay-Lyons, M., & Eskes, G. (2020). Effects of exercise on cognitive performance in older adults: A narrative review of the evidence, possible biological mechanisms, and recommendations for exercise prescription. *Journal of Aging Research, 2020*, 1407896. https://doi.org/10.1155/2020/1407896

Thomas, B. P., Tarumi, T., Sheng, M., Tseng, B., Womack, K. B., Cullum, C. M., Rypma, B., Zhang, R., & Lu, H. (2020). Brain perfusion change in patients with mild cognitive impairment after 12 months of aerobic exercise training. *Journal of Alzheimer's Disease, 75*(2), 617–631. https://doi.org/10.3233/JAD-190977

Wilckens, K. A., Stillman, C. M., Waiwood, A. M., Kang, C., Leckie, R. L., Peven, J. C., Foust, J. E., Fraundorf, S. H., & Erickson, K. I. (2021).

Exercise interventions preserve hippocampal volume: A meta-analysis. *Hippocampus, 31*(3), 335–347. https://doi.org/10.1002/hipo.23292

World Health Organization. (2020). *WHO guidelines on physical activity and sedentary behaviour.*

Yue, C., Yu, Q., Zhang, Y., Herold, F., Mei, J., Kong, Z., Perrey, S., Liu, J., Müller, N. G., Zhang, Z., Tao, Y., Kramer, A., Becker, B., & Zou, L. (2020). Regular Tai Chi practice is associated with improved memory as well as structural and functional alterations of the hippocampus in the elderly. *Frontiers in Aging Neuroscience, 12*, 586770. https://doi.org/10.3389/fnagi.2020.586770

# CHAPTER 3

# USE IT OR LOSE IT: MENTAL ACTIVITY FOR A HEALTHY BRAIN

I already have it figured out. In about 10 years, I want to learn a new language. I will probably choose Spanish because it would help me as a psychologist to serve the growing number of Spanish speakers in the United States. A few years after that, I hope to learn to play the piano. I have dreamed of playing the piano since I was a young child, but I never made time to take lessons. I think it's about time to live that dream! After I reach some satisfactory level of competence in piano playing, I'll take art classes. I love art! In my younger days, painting and drawing were a big part of my life, but I've lost the hobby over time. And finally, when I retire, I plan to take courses in cultural anthropology, literature, and philosophy through one of the many lifelong learning programs offered online.

Did you notice a common theme in all of my plans? They all involve learning something new! Each will require me to challenge my brain by getting out of my comfort zone and doing something different. I came up with this plan because all my research and other professional experiences have taught me that staying mentally active is an important key to lifelong brain health.

This chapter summarizes what scientists have discovered about the benefits to your brain that come with participating in cognitively stimulating activities throughout your life. You will learn what research tells us about online brain games that claim to be the answer to memory decline that can come with age. And we'll discuss ideas for challenging your brain in enjoyable ways through your hobbies and day-to-day activities.

## WHAT RESEARCH TELLS US

More than 2 centuries ago, Roman statesman, lawyer, and renowned orator Cicero wrote, "Old men retain their intellects well enough, if only they keep their minds active and fully employed." This astute remark captures in a nutshell what modern science tells us: By keeping an active mind throughout life, we can maintain a healthier brain as we grow older.

### Early Mental Stimulation Builds the Foundation for a Healthier Brain Later in Life

The mid-1990s saw the launch of two companies that quickly became popular with new parents: the Baby Einstein Company and Leapfrog Enterprises. Both companies are premised on the idea that infants and toddlers develop better if they are exposed to stimulating toys, videos, and games. Despite inconsistent scientific evidence that any particular product affects early childhood development, there *is* good evidence that we get a brain boost when we are exposed to stimulating environments, even as early as infancy. Healthy brains develop over time, starting with the earliest stages of life.

For example, researchers at the Cincinnati Children's Hospital published a study in 2020 that showed remarkable differences in preschoolers' brains based on how often their caregivers read to them. A group of children between 3 and 5 years old received a special type of brain scan that allows researchers to measure the health of white matter in the brain. White matter is made up of bundles or tracts of fibers that connect brain cells to each other and to the rest of the nervous system. These connections make it possible for the brain to communicate across different areas, a process necessary for the brain to function well. The researchers also asked a parent of each tyke to complete a questionnaire about how often they read to the child and what type of books they read. The children who were read to the most had the healthiest white matter tracts in areas of the brain that support language and reading skills. To top it off, they also performed better on vocabulary, language, and reading tests.

Early childhood is a critical period that lays the foundation for the rest of development. Exposing ourselves to mentally stimulating environments in adolescence, adulthood, and late life is critical to building upon that foundation to support a healthy brain. Of all the ways that early life mental stimulation affects brain health throughout life, educational and occupational experiences top the list. People who are highly educated and people who have cognitively demanding jobs—jobs that require continual learning, problem solving, or critical thinking—tend to develop complex and efficient brains. As they grow older, this allows them to compensate for brain changes that often come with aging, maintaining their memory and cognitive abilities much longer than people with the same degree of brain damage who have not had as much mental stimulation. Psychologists and neuroscientists use the term "cognitive reserve" for this buffer against brain changes.

During my time as a postdoctoral fellow in a laboratory at the National Institute on Aging, I witnessed remarkable examples of cognitive reserve. Since the 1950s, this lab has been conducting a study called the Baltimore Longitudinal Study of Aging, or BLSA. Remember from Chapter 1 that longitudinal studies follow the same people over time to capture *changes*, not just differences, in their functioning. BLSA participants complete questionnaires, take cognitive tests, and receive a host of medical assessments every year. Some agree to donate their brains to the study after death so researchers can answer important questions by examining brain tissue post-mortem. Over the course of my 3 years as a postdoctoral fellow, I was part of a team that met once a year to look at all of the cognitive test data for people in the study who had died that year. On the basis of their pattern of scores on memory and cognitive tests when they were alive, we would decide whether or not we thought they met criteria for Alzheimer's disease or another type of dementia. After we made that decision, a neuropathologist—a doctor who specializes in diagnosing brain diseases by examining brain tissue under a microscope—would reveal the results of his examination.

On multiple occasions, we looked at a BLSA participant's cognitive test scores and found that they were doing remarkably well, even into their 80s or 90s! We determined that they did not have any type of dementia because their cognitive functioning had been stable over the years, in contrast to the pattern of progressive decline that we usually see in dementia. In some cases, though, the neuropathologist would report on his findings and, shockingly, the participant's brain was full of the plaques and tangles that we find in people with Alzheimer's disease. How were these individuals able to function so well while they were alive despite the massive changes to their brain? This is where cognitive reserve comes in. Many BLSA participants had advanced degrees and worked as doctors, lawyers, professors, or judges. In other words, they had a lifetime of continual mental stimulation through their education and occupations. What we do throughout our lifetime can build cognitive reserve.

## Mentally Engaging Activities in Your Senior Years Can Give Your Brain a Boost

As a professor at Georgia State University, an urban university in downtown Atlanta, I have the pleasure of teaching an incredibly diverse group of students from every walk of life, cultural background, and age. I recently taught a small master's-level class that included a woman named Amy, who was taking advantage of Georgia State's GSU-62 program, which provides tuition waivers for students aged 62 and over. I found it thrilling and inspiring to witness her dedication to lifelong learning. I immediately thought of her when I started writing this chapter, so I asked her if she would explain what motivated her to stay mentally active in her senior years.

At the age of 73, Amy is working on a master's degree in gerontology. She described this as her most recent accomplishment in a life filled with learning. When she was younger, she earned a bachelor's degree in French and a master's degree in taxation, which boosted her career as a certified public accountant. Moved by an acute reminder of life's brevity and fragility after the death of her parents, Amy developed a small accounting business that specialized in services for older adults. A vision she had of offering financial planning for older adults and support for those facing tough decisions at the end of life motivated her to pursue a master's degree in gerontology.

When I asked her what she found most rewarding about going back to school, Amy exclaimed, "This experience has brought so much joy into my life!" She said that being in school at her age had increased the diversity in her social circle and introduced her to many people with a passion for social service and justice. She felt welcomed as a student and has not met any ageist stereotypes, a fear that sometimes deters seniors from embarking on learning experiences with younger students. She sees herself as a valuable part of the university community.

I enjoyed learning about Amy's activities outside of the classroom that helped keep her mind engaged. Over the years, she has been active in her church and served on the board of her homeowners' association. She also practices textile arts. She said that she is "continually learning new techniques for quilting and knitting, exploring the edge of what's just beyond [her] skill level."

Notice that Amy is staying cognitively engaged both through a formal educational program and mentally stimulating hobbies. Research shows us that both types of activities support a healthy brain. One study followed a group of more than 400 retired older adults for about 14 years, on average, gathering data every few years. The researchers asked participants about their primary occupations when they were younger, including the complexity of their jobs, such as how often they had to process information, manage or mentor people, or work with machinery. The participants also answered questions about their leisure activities during older adulthood, and they completed cognitive tests. It turned out that both job complexity in earlier adulthood and leisure activity later in life protected memory and cognitive ability. Those who had greater job complexity fared better, as did those who regularly participated in cognitive activities (e.g., reading books, or playing puzzles or chess) or physical activities (e.g., sports and walks).

One of the great things about keeping your mind engaged through leisure activities is that it is never too late to start! You might not get excited about the idea of going back to school in your 70s, as Amy did, but you might find it compelling to pick up a new hobby that challenges your brain. And the good news is that you can benefit from keeping your mind active at any age, even if you didn't go far in school or have a mentally challenging job in your younger years. In a recent study, people over age 60 were given cognitive tests and questionnaires about their education, work history, and leisure activities, similar to the study just described. The people with less formal education got the biggest boost in cognitive functioning from participating in mentally engaging activities, such as volunteering in their free time.

Mentally engaging leisure activities can be especially important in retirement, when we lose the regular cognitive stimulation that comes from working outside of the home. Studies show that many people experience a decline in their cognitive skills after retirement, but retired people who stay mentally active have less decline. Staying active can also help us maintain a sense of purpose after retirement, which fosters a sense of well-being.

Research tells us that changes in the brain might explain the cognitive boost we get from having mentally stimulating hobbies. People who regularly read the newspaper, write letters, visit a library, attend a play, or play games such as chess or checkers have healthier white matter—the tracts that connect different parts of the brain—compared with people who rarely or never take part in meaningful and stimulating activities. Studies also show that playing an instrument and singing increase the size of brain structures that are important for healthy cognitive functioning, such as the hippocampus and frontal lobes.

## People With Dementia Fare Better if They Stay Mentally Engaged

What if you or your loved one has dementia? It's not too late to benefit from staying mentally active! You may have noticed the variety of activities that senior centers, assisted living facilities, and nursing homes offer to clients and residents. Board games, dance classes, arts and crafts sessions, writing groups, and many other activities keep the wheels turning, even in people who experience the ravages of dementia and other neurological disorders on brain functioning. People in the later stages of dementia might find these types of activities to be too challenging, which can lead to distress. But activities such as looking at old family pictures and reminiscing, or even everyday activities, such as folding towels, can be mentally stimulating for people with advanced dementia. Cognitive stimulation is one way that people with dementia can potentially slow down memory and cognitive decline, making it more likely that they can maintain everyday functioning longer.

Mental activity not only capitalizes on the cognitive skills that people with dementia have been able to retain, it can also strengthen some of the skills that have started to decline. Keep in mind that people with dementia typically maintain some of their cognitive skills for years after their diagnosis. As we learned in Chapter 1, there are different causes of dementia, and each cause progresses in a unique manner in the brain. Because of this, cognitive impairment in different types of dementia follows different courses. For example, someone with dementia caused by Alzheimer's disease is likely to quickly forget recent information, such as details of a conversation they had the night before, and they may struggle to think of words that are on the tip of their tongue. On the other hand, someone with dementia caused by damage to the blood vessels in their brain is likely to have problems focusing their attention on a television show or news story, and they might need extra time to mentally process the world around them. What this means is that not all cognitive abilities decline right away in dementia, which allows people with dementia to capitalize on their stronger cognitive skills to actively participate in pastimes that keep their minds engaged.

Longitudinal research—the kind that tracks the same people over time—shows that a high level of cognitive activity later in life is associated with a nearly 50% reduced risk of developing dementia 4 to 5 years later. In people who already have dementia, mentally stimulating activities improve memory and cognitive test scores. Studies also show benefits on the mood, overall well-being, and communication abilities of people with dementia. It is worth noting that the boost in memory and cognitive abilities tends to be fairly small. This means that you should not expect someone with dementia to have dramatic improvements in their functioning if they become more mentally active. Still, even small gains can be meaningful for a person and their family in the midst of a progressive disease.

## Cognitive Training Can Improve Functioning and Delay Decline

Another way to challenge your brain comes from *cognitive training*. As the term implies, compared with mentally challenging hobbies and other leisure activities, cognitive training is a more structured, organized approach to engaging your brain. It involves guided practice on a set of tasks designed to improve particular cognitive skills, such as memory or attention. The training can be done on a one-one-basis or in small groups, and these days it is usually computerized. An example of cognitive training would be if you worked with a neuro-psychologist to learn how to better solve problems that require you to identify the pattern in a series of letters or numbers on a computer screen. The neuropsychologist could teach you strategies to identify a pattern and have you practice the strategies daily using a series of mental exercises that require you to use your reasoning and problem-solving skills. Clearly this is a much more formal way of using your brain than reading a book or playing chess, but all of these activities keep your mind active!

Computerized cognitive training was the focus of the ACTIVE study. ACTIVE stands for Advanced Cognitive Training for Independent and Vital Elderly, capturing the study's purpose—to determine whether cognitive training can improve cognitive abilities and, as a result, help people 65 and older preserve their ability to independently perform day-to-day activities, such as driving or managing their medications. This impressive study followed more than 2,800 seniors for 10 years, comparing research volunteers who were randomly placed either into one of three different cognitive training groups or into a control group that did not receive any training. Remember from Chapter 1 that this study design means it is an intervention study.

ACTIVE study volunteers assigned to one of the training groups spent 5 weeks completing up to 10 weekly sessions of computerized training. Each person was assigned to a training group that focused on improving either memory, reasoning skills (the ability to solve problems involving patterns or rules), or their speed of processing of visual information presented on a computer screen. Some volunteers completed one round of training, and others completed an additional round or two of training, called "booster sessions." Three main break-through scientific findings came out of this study.

First, each type of training led to better performance on cognitive tests that relied on the same abilities—so people who received memory training scored better on other memory tests, and so on. Even more impressive, the cognitive boost from the reasoning training and the speed-of-processing training lasted for 10 years! The people who had booster sessions saw even more of a boost to their cognitive skills.

Second, when the researchers followed the volunteers from time to time during the 10 years of the study, they noted that people who received cognitive training had fewer problems with day-to-day activities necessary to live independently, like housework, shopping, cooking, driving, or managing money. This is important because people who have problems with these everyday tasks are more likely to move into an assisted living facility or nursing home, or to require help from family or professionals.

The third major finding from the ACTIVE study was that people who received cognitive training were less likely to develop dementia over the 10-year period of the study. For example, the volunteers who received 11 to 14 sessions of speed-of-processing training were 48% less likely to develop dementia compared with the control group! The study also found that more doses of the speed-of-processing training delayed onset of dementia, meaning that, among volunteers who developed dementia, those who had received the speed-of-processing training had more healthy years before their dementia took hold.

The ACTIVE Study is the largest of its kind, but there are other research studies that point in the same direction. Not all studies report consistent findings, but overall the majority of them show that cognitive training can lead to modest gains in cognitive function in healthy middle-aged and older adults and in people who have already started to experience some cognitive decline. And this seems to be rooted in changes to the brain. Cognitive training changes brain structure, such as the white matter tracts we discussed earlier, and brain function, such as the blood flow patterns when the brain is at work.

## What About Those "Brain Games" We Hear All About?

An important word of warning here is warranted: Cognitive training is not the same as the commercially available "brain games" that often make grandiose claims about making you smarter, improving your attention, and protecting your memory from decline. What makes these claims grandiose is that scientific studies of these types of brain fitness games have not produced any convincing evidence that they work. In fact, the creators and marketers of the popular Lumosity "brain training" program paid millions of dollars in a settlement with the Federal Trade Commission in response to charges that they deceived consumers with unfounded claims that their product could improve cognition, treat symptoms of attention-deficit/hyperactivity disorder, and boost school and work performance.

Experts from the Global Council on Brain Health, a group of scientists, doctors, and policy experts around the world who specialize in brain health, described the evidence supporting the benefits of commercial brain games as "weak to nonexistent." They concluded that even though playing such games might help you get better at that particular game, there isn't enough evidence that you will see improvements in everyday functioning. One of the problems seems to be that the difficulty level of commercial brain games is too low. To get the biggest boost to your functioning, your cognitive activities should challenge you, requiring you to work hard enough to feel some mental strain. Experts say that training programs should grow more challenging as your performance improves so that you have to keep pushing yourself. Commercial brain training programs also tend to miss three other characteristics experts say are important for the success of cognitive training: Training works better when it (a) is delivered in a group, (b) uses multiple cognitive strategies—such as using a combination of imagery and repetition to improve memory—and (c) is similar to the skills you use in everyday life.

What should you do when, on the one hand, studies have shown cognitive training can help improve and maintain a healthy brain, but on the other hand, the kinds of training programs you're most likely to come across have shown little evidence that they are effective? Consider these pointers:

- Before paying money for any brain training program, find out if there is any scientific evidence that the program is effective. It's not enough for the company's website to claim that they have done their own research and shown it to be effective. Ideally, the research will come from people outside of the company who aren't biased to say that the program works. I suggest feeling more cautious if only one study supports the program. Look for *replication*, which means that study results have been reproduced at least once by a separate study.
- You also want to know if any research findings have been published in a scientific journal. This means that the research has been peer reviewed—experts in the field have had a chance to take a look at the methods used, statistical analyses, and conclusions and deemed the research scientifically sound.
- Check to see if the company has a scientific advisory board. The board should include a group of experts in brain health whose

professional credentials are clearly spelled out on the company website so that you will know why they are considered experts in the field. A scientific advisory board helps to guide product development, playing an important role in making sure that the training program is backed by science. For example, members of the scientific advisory board for my company, CerebroFit, have expertise in areas such as cognitive aging, dementia prevention, brain health, and physical activity, which helps to ensure that all of our services promoting brain health are grounded in the latest research findings.

Even with these pieces of advice to help you evaluate brain training programs, my professional opinion is that, overall, you are better off doing any brain training program under the care of a neuropsychologist. Some insurance providers cover brain training, which is often referred to as "cognitive rehabilitation" in cases where the goal is to improve functioning in someone with a condition such as dementia, stroke, or head injury. Cognitive rehabilitation has the benefit of using an individualized approach, tailoring the treatment to the person's needs.

Ultimately, your best bet is to incorporate a variety of mentally engaging activities into your life, including your hobbies and social activities. So let's start planning your mentally active life!

## ENGAGE YOUR BRAIN! PLANNING FOR YOUR MENTALLY ACTIVE LIFE

Katherine Johnson was the NASA mathematician and aerospace pioneer portrayed in the book and film *Hidden Figures*. This trail-blazing Black woman persevered through racism and sexism and made her mark on history. She performed the calculations that led to the success of multiple NASA missions, including John Glenn's historic Friendship 7 mission in 1962, which made him the first American to orbit the earth. Johnson lived to be 101! A *Forbes* article described her as a "lifelong learner." A lover of travel and card games, she once told an interviewer, "You lose your curiosity when you stop learning."

Similarly, Pablo Picasso famously remained prolific in his senior years. Architects in the city of Chicago commissioned him to create a public sculpture in 1963—at the age of 82! This work, completed 3 years later, was not his only product as an octogenarian. He tirelessly created works of art from 1968 to 1971, well beyond the time in life that we associate with retiring and slowing down. In fact, he created more art in the 4 years before he died than in any other 4-year period in his life. This masterful artist continued to explore different painting styles, forms of artwork, and materials until his death at the age of 91, even creating his first etchings and engravings in his final years.

Johnson and Picasso both exemplify a key characteristic of the group of seniors dubbed "SuperAgers" by neurologist Marsel Mesulam: They continue to embrace mental challenges as they age. SuperAgers maintain their cognitive abilities into their 80s and 90s, performing as well as, or even better than, their younger counterparts on tests of memory and cognitive functioning. This exceptional group also shows fewer signs of change in their brains related to age, such as volume loss. We don't know for sure if habits such as taking on challenges, socializing, and staying physically active directly *cause* SuperAgers to age well. It's possible that genes, or other life experiences are at play. But we do know that intervention studies support the link between mental activity and healthy brains later in life. Studies show a boost in different measures of brain health—such as cognitive test performance and brain functioning—in adults who participate in mentally engaging activities. These are compelling reasons to stay mentally active!

Members of the Global Council on Brain Health have come to the consensus that cognitively stimulating activities influence how well your brain functions. They outlined recommendations for people to challenge their brains at any age. They suggest that people start a mentally active lifestyle as soon as possible, regardless of age. Let's go over some guidelines for incorporating cognitively stimulating activities into your lifestyle.

| Cognitive Stimulation Tips | | |
|---|---|---|
| Find new ways to stimulate your brain | Engage your brain along with someone else | Choose an activity that you enjoy |
| Make it easy on yourself | Aim for purposeful (deliberate) practice | Find an activity where someone will notice whether you are present |
| Use life stages and transitions to change things up | Study something you are interested in | Choose activities involving both mental and physical engagement |

*Note.* From "Engage Your Brain: GCBH Recommendations on Cognitively Stimulating Activities," July 2017 (https://www.aarp.org/content/dam/aarp/health/brain_health/2017/07/gcbh-cognitively-stimulating-activities-report-english-aarp.doi.10.26419%252Fpia.00001.001.pdf). Copyright 2017 by the Global Council on Brain Health. Adapted with permission.

## Break Out of Your Daily Routine

It's human nature to get into a routine and then default to that routine. When it comes to brain health, though, what we need the most is to challenge our brain in new ways. Experts recommend that people incorporate cognitively stimulating activities into their lifestyle that are novel, highly engaging, mentally challenging, and fun.

The good thing about planning for a mentally active lifestyle is that you have so many choices! Activities that you do regularly can be cognitively stimulating if they involve the characteristics named above. Mental activity comes in many forms, so be flexible in choosing activities that challenge your thinking. We don't have good evidence that one particular cognitively stimulating activity is more effective than another at maintaining your brain health, so the key is variety. It's important to seek out new sources of stimulation regardless of whether you're already participating in mentally engaging activities. Start by adding one or two new activities into your life.

Use the "Brainstorming Enjoyable Cognitively Stimulating Activities" worksheet (Exhibit 3.1) to brainstorm ideas for enjoyable activities that can keep your mind stimulated. Think about different types of activities. For example, a new hobby might be doing arts and crafts. Something new you would like to learn could be playing the guitar or learning American Sign Language. Or you might make a point to spend more time going to museums or following the stock market. Similar to what you did for brainstorming physical activities in Chapter 2, think about any barriers that might make it hard for you to take up the mentally stimulating activities you want to pursue. Consider whether you have any resources to help you get past those barriers. For example, if you're interested in museums but transportation is a barrier, you might look for virtual exhibits available online. Think outside the box, and ask your friends and family for ideas too.

## EXHIBIT 3.1. Brainstorming Enjoyable Cognitively Stimulating Activities

| Old Hobbies to Resume | What Are the Barriers? | What Resources Will Help? |
| --- | --- | --- |
| | | |
| | | |
| | | |
| | | |

| New Hobbies I Would Like to Try | What Are the Barriers? | What Resources Will Help? |
| --- | --- | --- |
| | | |
| | | |
| | | |
| | | |

| New Things I Would Like to Learn | What Are the Barriers? | What Resources Will Help? |
| --- | --- | --- |
| | | |
| | | |
| | | |
| | | |

| Other Activities I Find Interesting | What Are the Barriers? | What Resources Will Help? |
| --- | --- | --- |
| | | |
| | | |
| | | |
| | | |

---

### IDEAS FOR MENTAL ACTIVITY

- Practice arts and crafts
- Read a book, magazine, or newspaper
- Attend church activities
- Collect stamps or other items
- Take a course
- Play cards, chess, or other board games
- Cook something new or take a cooking class
- Pursue cultural or political interests
- Garden
- Investigate your genealogy
- Join a social group
- Follow the stock market or manage investments
- Practice tai chi
- Teach someone a skill
- Learn a new technology

- Join a theater group or go to the theater
- Play with your children or grandchildren
- Make complex home repairs
- Learn to juggle
- Learn a new language
- Go to the library
- Learn how to play a musical instrument
- Go to a museum
- Take photography classes
- Listen to a podcast or radio show
- Plan a family event or vacation
- Do crossword puzzles or jigsaw puzzles
- Watch TV or listen to music
- Travel
- Play trivia games
- Volunteer in your community
- Write a letter, poem, or story

## Embrace Mental Challenges

Get out of your comfort zone and challenge yourself to learn something new! This might feel strenuous at times, which can be unpleasant. For example, I might get frustrated when I face the challenge of learning to read music once I start taking piano lessons. But this

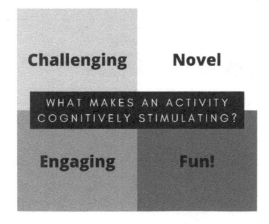

Challenging    Novel

WHAT MAKES AN ACTIVITY
COGNITIVELY STIMULATING?

Engaging    Fun!

strain is a good thing, similar to the good that can come from running an extra lap even after your body is exhausted. To reap the greatest rewards, we must push past the discomfort that inevitably comes from challenging ourselves. Patience and perseverance are essential. At the same time, it is important to choose activities that you enjoy so that you will stay motivated to continue.

## Tips for Success

Set yourself up for success by doing what you enjoy, by choosing activities that are novel, challenging, engaging, and fun, and by keeping a positive mindset.

### Do What You Enjoy

The best way to make sure that your cognitively stimulating activities become a part of your lifestyle, rather than just a phase, is to choose activities that you find interesting and enjoyable. Are there things you always wanted to try but never got around to? Maybe now is the time to go for it. Are there old hobbies or intellectual pursuits that you gave up? Consider resuming them. Start by finding two or three activities that you *want* to pursue and that don't feel like a chore. You want to make sure the activity challenges you, but you don't want the occasional frustration that comes from getting out of your comfort zone to ruin your enjoyment. As an example, think about the plans I described at the start of this chapter. I want to take piano lessons in my senior years because I've always had the interest but I never got around to it. I also want to take up artwork again; this is an example of revisiting an old activity. Both of these activities are motivating to me because I am very interested in them and enjoy art and music. At the same time, both will mentally challenge and engage me.

## Think Quality Over Quantity

More is not necessarily better when it comes to cognitively stimulating activities. The variety and quality of the activities are most important. The activities you choose should be novel, challenging, engaging, and fun. So if you have been doing Sudoku puzzles for years, simply putting more hours into Sudoku isn't your best option. Instead, you can try a new type of game or puzzle that challenges your mind in a different way and requires you to focus your attention and that you find enjoyable. Alternatively, you can do something completely different, such as taking an art class or learning how to juggle.

Consider activities that include a physical component or a social component. For example, tai chi includes a combination of slow-motion exercise and focused attention. Gardening requires planning, attention, and memory, but it is also a good way to introduce more physical activity into your life. You can bring in a social aspect by participating in group activities, such as a book club or art class. Play games with your grandchildren to get the triple benefit of mental activity, social activity, and emotional fulfillment. Studies show that incorporating a sense of purpose or meaning in your activities can benefit brain health. Volunteering might provide that sense of purpose while also keeping your mind active and giving you a social outlet. We will talk more about social engagement in Chapter 4.

## Remember That Mindset Matters

Popular culture is full of stereotypes about aging that are not true, or are only partially true. A common fallacy is "You can't teach an old dog new tricks." This old saying comes from the incorrect assumption that as we get older, we cannot learn anything new. This is not true at all! One of the problems with myths like this is that they perpetuate negative stereotypes, and, over time, many of us internalize those stereotypes. Then we worry about confirming stereotypes, and our decisions and behavior may be affected.

Psychologists use the term "stereotype threat" to describe the fear of confirming a negative stereotype about our group. We see this, for example, when girls perform worse on math tests compared with boys if they are reminded before the test of the stereotype that males have better math skills than females. My colleague at Georgia State University, Sarah Barber, is an expert on stereotype threat in older adults. This is how she described the phenomenon:

> When older people are asked to take a test assessing their cogni-tive abilities in a research lab, or in a medical clinic, they may feel anxious or concerned about why they are being evaluated. They may also worry that the researcher or physician expects them to do poorly because of their age. These concerns can sometimes lead people to do worse than their potential. (personal communication, October 27, 2020)

Barber's research team uses innovative techniques to study stereotype threat. For example, they might give a memory test to a group of older adults and manipulate the test instructions to evoke stereotype threat in half of their participants. They tell research volun-teers in the stereotype-threat condition that the purpose of the study is to compare the memory abilities of younger and older adults and that they are part of the older adult group. In contrast, they may simply tell the other half of their volunteers that they are examining individual differences in memory abilities, without mentioning age comparisons at all—this is the *control* condition. Barber explained that in studies like this, they usually find that volunteers perform more poorly on the memory test when they receive the stereotype-threat instructions compared with the control instructions.

How does this relate to our goal of maintaining a mentally active life? Stereotype threat can take away our confidence about our cognitive abilities and thus can make us feel less motivated to try a difficult new cognitive task, such as learning a new language or taking a course. To overcome possible feelings of stereotype threat, Barber suggested that you try to think of reasons besides your age that might explain why a task is difficult. For example, maybe you're tired that day. Or maybe the task is difficult for younger people too. "Try to avoid making . . . age-based attributions!" she said. Barber advised that you shift your mindset: Interpret the situation as a challenge that you can overcome rather than as a threat that will hinder your performance.

Your attitude plays an important role in your journey to a healthier brain. Don't let your age, past experiences, or current barriers put you in a pessimistic mindset. Remember that it is never too late to start a mentally active life, regardless of your lifestyle in the past. You or your loved ones can also stay mentally active even while experiencing memory or cognitive decline, or if one of you have Alzheimer's disease or another type of dementia. Also, similar to what we discussed for physical activity, you can brainstorm ways of overcoming barriers to engaging in cognitively stimulating activities.

## SUMMARY

To wrap up, remember these key points:

- Research studies show that being mentally active is an important key to lifelong brain health.
- What you do throughout your life matters. Experiences earlier in life, such as how far you go in school and the quality of your educational experiences, can put you on the road to a healthy brain later in life. But what you do later in life matters, too—such as continuing to participate in cognitively stimulating activities in your later years.
- Staying mentally engaged throughout your life can reduce your risk of dementia. For those who have already developed

dementia, mental stimulation is important for helping slow down memory and cognitive decline.

- Formal cognitive training can improve cognitive abilities, but the benefits are usually specific to the particular ability that is trained. Cognitive training is best done with a neuropsychologist who can tailor the training to your needs.
- There is little evidence that brain games, such as the ones offered online, have any substantial benefit on the brain. Instead, focus on adding novel activities into your life that engage your brain, challenge you, and are enjoyable.
- Embrace mental challenges. A little bit of strain goes a long way in boosting the health of your brain. Consider activities that include a physical component or a social component to get an even greater boost.
- Let go of stereotypes about aging. You can stay mentally engaged regardless of your age, history, or mental abilities.

## RESOURCES AND SUGGESTED READINGS

**Global Council on Brain Health, "Engage Your Brain"**: https://www.aarp.org/content/dam/aarp/health/brain_health/2017/07/gcbh-cognitively-stimulating-activities-report-english-aarp.doi.10.26419%252Fpia.00001.001.pdf
Science-based recommendations for staying mentally active to achieve a healthy brain.

**Global Council on Brain Health, "Music on Our Minds"**: https://www.aarp.org/content/dam/aarp/health/brain_health/2020/06/gcbh-music-report-english.doi.10.26419-2Fpia.00103.001.pdf
Science-based recommendations for boosting brain health and mental well-being through music.

**Golden Carers, "Activities for Seniors":** https://www.goldencarers.com/activities/

Website with thousands of activity ideas that cover a range of interests to keep you and your loved one mentally engaged. Includes monthly calendars with activity ideas that go along with events and celebrations, plus other resources to get you organized.

Powell, T. (2017). *The brain injury workbook: Exercises for cognitive rehabilitation* (2nd ed.). Routledge.

Information, exercises, and handouts to help people with head injuries improve their memory, executive functions, and emotional adjustment.

Bourne, L. E., & Healy, A. F. (2014). *Train your mind for peak performance: A science-based approach for achieving your goals*. American Psychological Association.

Tools from cognitive psychologists to help you maximize your ability to learn new information or skills. Perfect as you take on new hobbies and activities to stay mentally engaged!

**AARP Learning Academy:** https://www.aarp.org/academy

Lots of resources to keep you learning throughout your life, including links to online and in-person workshops about a variety of topics for seniors and for caregivers.

**FutureLearn:** https://www.futurelearn.com/

Free online courses, related to career fields or hobbies and personal interests, that you can take at your own pace.

**Coursera:** https://www.coursera.org/

Free online courses, all linked to well-established universities and taught by professionals in the specific field. Includes readings, videos, and short assessments.

## SELECTED REFERENCES

Alvares Pereira, G., Silva Nunes, M. V., Alzola, P., & Contador, I. (2021). Cognitive reserve and brain maintenance in aging and dementia: An integrative review. *Applied Neuropsychology: Adult*. Advance online publication. https://doi.org/10.1080/23279095.2021.1872079

Andel, R., Finkel, D., & Pedersen, N. L. (2016). Effects of preretirement work complexity and postretirement leisure activity on cognitive aging. *Journals of Gerontology: Series B. Psychological Sciences and Social Sciences*, 71(5), 849–856. https://doi.org/10.1093/geronb/gbv026

Arfanakis, K., Wilson, R. S., Barth, C. M., Capuano, A. W., Vasireddi, A., Zhang, S., Fleischman, D. A., & Bennett, D. A. (2016). Cognitive activity, cognitive function, and brain diffusion characteristics in old age. *Brain Imaging and Behavior*, 10(2), 455–463. https://doi.org/10.1007/s11682-015-9405-5

Barber, S. J. (2017). An examination of age-based stereotype threat about cognitive decline. *Perspectives on Psychological Science*, 12(1), 62–90. https://doi.org/10.1177/1745691616656345

Carbone, E., Gardini, S., Pastore, M., Piras, F., Vincenzi, M., & Borella, E. (2021). Cognitive Stimulation Therapy (CST) for older adults with mild-to-moderate dementia in Italy: Effects on cognitive functioning and on emotional and neuropsychiatric symptoms. *Journals of Gerontology: Series B. Psychological Sciences and Social Sciences*. Advance online publication. https://doi.org/10.1093/geronb/gbab007

Fan, B. J. Y., & Wong, R. Y. M. (2019). Effect of cognitive training on daily function in older people without major neurocognitive disorder: A systematic review. *Geriatrics*, 4(3), 44. https://doi.org/10.3390/geriatrics4030044

Gibbor, L., Forde, L., Yates, L., Orfanos, S., Komodromos, C., Page, H., Harvey, K., & Spector, A. (2021). A feasibility randomised control trial of individual cognitive stimulation therapy for dementia: Impact on cognition, quality of life and positive psychology. *Aging and Mental Health*, 25(6), 999–1007. https://doi.org/10.1080/13607863.2020.1747048

Hu, M., Wu, X., Shu, X., Hu, H., Chen, Q., Peng, L., & Feng, H. (2021). Effects of computerised cognitive training on cognitive impairment:

A meta-analysis. *Journal of Neurology, 268*(5), 1680–1688. https://doi.org/10.1007/s00415-019-09522-7

Hutton, J. S., Dudley, J., Horowitz-Kraus, T., DeWitt, T., & Holland, S. K. (2020). Associations between home literacy environment, brain white matter integrity and cognitive abilities in preschool-age children. *Acta Paediatrica, 109*(7), 1376–1386. https://doi.org/10.1111/apa.15124

Lee, Y., Chi, I., & Palinkas, L. A. (2019). Retirement, leisure activity engagement, and cognition among older adults in the United States. *Journal of Aging and Health, 31*(7), 1212–1234. https://doi.org/10.1177/0898264318767030

O'Brien, R. J., Resnick, S. M., Zonderman, A. B., Ferrucci, L., Crain, B. J., Pletnikova, O., Rudow, G., Iacono, D., Riudavets, M. A., Driscoll, I., Price, D. L., Martin, L. J., & Troncoso, J. C. (2009). Neuropathologic studies of the Baltimore Longitudinal Study of Aging (BLSA). *Journal of Alzheimer's Disease, 18*(3), 665–675. https://doi.org/10.3233/JAD-2009-1179

Oveisgharan, S., Wilson, R. S., Yu, L., Schneider, J. A., & Bennett, D. A. (2020). Association of early-life cognitive enrichment with Alzheimer disease pathological changes and cognitive decline. *JAMA Neurology, 77*(10), 1217–1224. https://doi.org/10.1001/jamaneurol.2020.1941

Rebok, G. W., Ball, K., Guey, L. T., Jones, R. N., Kim, H. Y., King, J. W., Marsiske, M., Morris, J. N., Tennstedt, S. L., Unverzagt, F. W., & Willis, S. L. (2014). Ten-year effects of the Advanced Cognitive Training for Independent and Vital Elderly cognitive training trial on cognition and everyday functioning in older adults. *Journal of the American Geriatrics Society, 62*(1), 16–24. https://doi.org/10.1111/jgs.12607

Sarkamo, T. (2018). Music for the ageing brain: Cognitive, emotional, social, and neural benefits of musical leisure activities in stroke and dementia. *Dementia, 17*(6), 670–685. https://doi.org/10.1177/1471301217729237

Ten Brinke, L. F., Davis, J. C., Barha, C. K., & Liu-Ambrose, T. (2017). Effects of computerized cognitive training on neuroimaging outcomes in older adults: A systematic review. *BMC Geriatrics, 17*(1), 139. https://doi.org/10.1186/s12877-017-0529-x

Topiwala, H., Terrera, G. M., Stirland, L., Saunderson, K., Russ, T. C., Dozier, M. F., & Ritchie, C. W. (2018). Lifestyle and neurodegeneration in midlife as expressed on functional magnetic resonance imaging: A systematic review. *Alzheimer's & Dementia: Translational Research & Clinical Interventions*, 4, 182–194. https://doi.org/10.1016/j.trci. 2018.04.001

van Balkom, T. D., van den Heuvel, O. A., Berendse, H. W., van der Werf, Y. D., & Vriend, C. (2020). The effects of cognitive training on brain network activity and connectivity in aging and neurodegenerative diseases: A systematic review. *Neuropsychology Review*, *30*(2), 267–286. https://doi.org/10.1007/s11065-020-09440-w

Wassenaar, T. M., Yaffe, K., van der Werf, Y. D., & Sexton, C. E. (2019). Associations between modifiable risk factors and white matter of the aging brain: Insights from diffusion tensor imaging studies. *Neurobiology of Aging*, *80*, 56–70. https://doi.org/10.1016/j.neurobiolaging. 2019.04.006

# CHAPTER 4

# STAY CONNECTED: SOCIAL ACTIVITY FOR A HEALTHY BRAIN

The COVID-19 pandemic changed social interactions across the globe in ways that will undoubtedly affect us for years to come. I wrote most of this book from my home office as I hunkered down in a new world of near-isolation, trying to protect myself and those around me and help curb the pandemic by socially distancing. I miss going to cultural and sporting events with my husband, visiting my extended family, vacationing with my friends, and interacting with my colleagues during the work day. Even the term "social distancing" sounds ominous to me, an extrovert who relishes social interactions and a neuropsychologist who is well aware of the scientific link between social connectedness and health.

As the pandemic spread across the United States in March and April of 2020, more and more cities issued stay-at-home orders, and all of us found ourselves in uncharted territory. Not surprisingly, it didn't take long for news stories to emerge with headlines such as "Can We Conquer Loneliness in a Time of Social Isolation?" and "How to Manage Your Loneliness." Surveys showed that as many as one third of respondents reported feeling lonely because of the pandemic. Reports referred to a "loneliness epidemic." People became aware of the plethora of research studies documenting the long-term effects of chronic loneliness at a time when most of the usual social outlets were unavailable. It has been a time that demands flexibility, resilience, and creativity to maintain our well-being.

I hope that the pandemic has driven the message home that social disconnectedness has a number of ill effects. Equally important, the reverse is also true when it comes to maintaining a healthy brain: Maintaining a strong social network and engaging in regular social activity can positively affect your brain as you age and promote a sense of wellness throughout your life.

This chapter discusses the importance of social connections for brain health. You will learn how social isolation and loneliness have a negative impact on the brain, while social engagement is linked to healthier brains, better cognitive functioning, and better mood. We will go over tips to help you add social activities to your life and strengthen your social network within the context of your personal preferences and circumstances.

## WHAT RESEARCH TELLS US

Humans are social by nature. Like other primates, we live in groups and have large, developed brains that enable us to manage the intricacies of social interactions. In fact, primates who have larger social group sizes also have larger brains. Although we might differ from each other in how much we seek out social connections, we share an intrinsic need to interact with other people. It's no wonder that many psychiatric disorders involve disruption to normal social behavior. For example, people with autism might have considerable trouble understanding social cues such as tone of voice or body language, and people with schizotypal personality disorder often have few, if any, close relationships. It is also unsurprising that an entire branch of science—the social sciences—focuses on human societies and social relationships. There is now a field of study called "social neuroscience" that examines how social experiences and behaviors affect, and are affected by, our brains.

The different social sciences focus on many aspects of social behavior, including *social engagement*, or how much we interact with others, take up purposeful activities with others, and maintain meaningful relationships. On the flip side, *social isolation* refers to an objective lack of social contact with others. Social engagement can promote social connection, a subjective feeling of being close and connected to other people, whereas social isolation can lead to loneliness, the subjective feeling of being isolated or alone. It's important to distinguish between the objective amount of contact we have with people versus the subjective feeling of being either connected or lonely, because not everyone desires the same amount of social contact. Loneliness occurs when there is a gap between the social engagement we want and the social engagement we have. Research tells us that social engagement can promote a healthy brain, whereas social isolation and loneliness can spell trouble for our brains.

## Social Disconnection Is Linked to Negative Brain Changes

I participated in a 2-day virtual workshop put on by the National Institute of Mental Health titled "Social Disconnection and Late-Life Suicide: Mechanisms, Treatment Targets, and Interventions During the Pandemic." Experts in neuroscience, geriatric psychiatry, epidemiology, and other health fields came together for a series of presentations and discussion groups via Zoom, all focused on understanding the current state of the science on social disconnection and how isolation relates to suicide in older adults. The workshop organizers asked me to moderate a roundtable discussion about the ways in which social isolation, brain changes, and cognitive changes relate to each other and increase the risk for suicidal thoughts and attempts.

The presentations and discussions over the course of the 2-day workshop summarized results from many different research studies showing that social isolation and loneliness are linked to negative changes in the brain. For example, Nancy Donovan, a researcher at Harvard, conducted a series of studies to examine the relationship between loneliness and markers of Alzheimer's disease. A group of senior volunteers answered three questions about loneliness: "How often do you feel that you lack companionship?" "How often do you feel left out?" and "How often do you feel isolated from others?" The volunteers chose from the options of "hardly ever," "some of the time," or "often" in answer to each question. The researchers also gave the volunteers special types of brain scans that showed the amount of *tau* and *amyloid beta*—the two primary markers of Alzheimer's disease—in their brains. The people who reported the most loneliness had more amyloid beta in their brains and also had more tau pathology in a part of the brain called the *entorhinal cortex*, an important hub in the brain's memory network. This is not the only study of its kind. Studies conducted by other researchers also have shown links between loneliness and changes in the size and function of the brain. This type of research tends to focus on older adults, but studies of young people have yielded similar findings: Loneliness is linked to negative changes in the brain.

The studies I just described used cross-sectional methods. You may recall that this means they show us relationships between two variables (such as loneliness and brain structure)—but they cannot tell us whether loneliness causes changes in brain health or vice versa. Longitudinal studies tackle the question of causality, and the results of many longitudinal studies support the idea that people who are socially isolated or lonely have more changes in brain health over time compared with their peers. One example comes from a study of more than 800 older adults who completed loneliness questionnaires and took tests of their cognitive skills at the start of the study as well as 1 year, 5 years, and 10 years after the study began. The people who reported the greatest loneliness not only had worse cognitive skills at the start of the study but also saw a decline over time in memory, perceptual speed, and spatial skills as well as a higher risk of developing Alzheimer's disease during the study.

Loneliness clearly has a detrimental impact on our brains. Fortunately, by increasing our social connectedness, we can combat loneliness and maintain a healthier brain.

## People Who Are Socially Connected Tend to Have Better Brain Health

Think about your social network. Do you have a large network that includes multiple family members and close friends, or a smaller network of just a few people? How much contact do you have with people in your network? How emotionally close do you feel with members of your network? Do you give or receive emotional support from your network? Does your experience with people in your network give you meaning or a sense of well-being? These are the kinds of questions researchers ask volunteers to get a sense of the quality of their social network. They can then relate network quality to data gathered about the structure or function of the brain, or about cognitive skills or other health measures. By and large, evidence from research studies suggests that quality of social networks and amount of social engagement are linked to healthier brains and better cognitive functioning. People who are socially engaged are better able to maintain their cognitive skills over the course of their lives and may experience slower cognitive decline later in life. Having a large social network, or one that provides a sense of well-being, satisfaction, and support, may offer protection against cognitive decline related to Alzheimer's disease pathology in the brain.

Again, keep in mind that studies that ask people about their social activities and link their responses to brain measures cannot conclusively tell us that social engagement directly improves or maintains brain health. This type of correlational analysis can tell us only that social engagement and brain health are related. But it is possible that people who already have healthy brains are the ones most likely to seek out social activity. This is where intervention studies are important. Remember that intervention studies are a special type of longitudinal study that systematically give volunteers some type of medical or psychological treatment for a period of time and then measure changes in functioning before and after the intervention. The results of intervention studies show the power of social engagement in promoting a healthy brain. They support the idea that social engagement causes improvement in brain health.

A few years ago, I found out about a fantastic program called Experience Corps (https://www.aarp.org/experience-corps/). This volunteer-based program matches adults over age 50 with kids who have difficulty reading. The program extensively trains volunteers so they can provide tutoring to struggling students, either one on one or in small groups. I immediately loved this idea when I heard about it, with its triple benefit of keeping seniors cognitively and socially engaged while benefiting kids and helping schools. I was even more impressed when I saw the data from research studies showing just how much the program benefited the brain health of the volunteers! Compared with people on a waiting list for the program, volunteers halted volume decline in regions of the brain that are vulnerable to dementia, and men were able to even reverse declines—some regions of their brains *increased* in size after 2 years of participating in the program! Volunteers' memory, processing speed, and reasoning skills improved, too.

## Social Activity Can Boost Mood, Too!

I will never forget the look of utter sadness on my 70-year-old client's face when she walked into the evaluation room with her daughter. She had come to see me for a neuropsychological evaluation because of the daughter's concerns about her memory, but what struck me the most was her depression. She had classic symptoms: She described herself as feeling "downhearted and sad" much of the time. She had lost interest in hobbies she used to enjoy, such as gardening and cooking. She was socially isolated, too. Her relationship with her husband was strained and was a source of anxiety rather than a fulfilling social connection. She occasionally spent time with her adult children and grandchildren, but as she became more depressed she became more and more withdrawn. With little motivation to do even basic self-care activities, such as getting out of bed and getting dressed, she felt little hope that her life would ever be fulfilling again.

Corroborated by her daughter, my client told me about the loss of memory and other cognitive problems she had been experiencing in recent months. She needed frequent reminders about her appointments and had trouble keeping up with a television show or news program, watching shows multiple times in an attempt to remember what she had seen and heard. Her mind wandered when she was cooking, causing her to forget ingredients in her recipes and to burn food after leaving it on the stove too long. She and her daughter were worried that these were all signs of Alzheimer's disease.

It is very common for me to see clients with a combination of memory complaints and depression. The relationship between brain health and depression is one of my areas of expertise, and in fact it is the focus of most of the research in my lab. Our studies, as well as studies from other researchers, show that depression is linked to many of the same brain regions that are important for healthy cognitive functioning. One example, the *prefrontal cortex*, lies at the very front of your brain. This area of the brain has a lot of different roles, thanks to its connection with so many other parts of the brain in what we call *neural networks* or *brain circuits*. Most relevant to my research, the prefrontal cortex helps us exert control over our emotional state—scientists call this *emotion regulation*. Regulating our emotions includes behaviors such as staying calm by reducing feelings of anger or anxiety, or focusing on reasons to feel happy.

In depression, the structure and function of the prefrontal cortex are altered, which helps explain the feelings of sadness that epitomize this common mental health condition. But we also know that changes in the prefrontal cortex are linked to problems with executive functions and other cognitive abilities. Remember that executive functions are a set of skills that we use to control and coordinate other cognitive abilities and behaviors, such as planning, organizing, and multitasking. All of this suggests that if certain parts of the brain, such as the prefrontal cortex, are disrupted, then depression and cognitive decline can both occur. It also follows that strategies that boost the health of the prefrontal cortex should benefit both your mood and your cognitive functioning. This indeed seems to be the case, and social engagement is one of those strategies! Studies show that when people are socially engaged, their mood is better. And we already learned that social engagement can improve cognitive functioning and change the brain. One of the brain regions that responds to social stimulation is the prefrontal cortex.

Let's go back to my client who was quite depressed and showing signs of cognitive decline. After putting together information from my clinical interview and her scores on a set of cognitive tests, my conclusion was that she did not have any signs of dementia; instead, her memory and attention lapses in day-to-day life were best explained by her depression. On the basis of what you've just learned, you might guess that one of my recommendations was for her to become more socially engaged.

Three months later, I was thrilled to receive a follow-up phone call from her daughter, filling me in on all the changes that had happened since her appointment. With help from their area agency on aging, my client was connected to a local senior center that offered quite a few opportunities to connect with other people, including group outings, arts and crafts, dance classes, exercise groups—you name it! The center provided transportation for her to attend three times a week, and she had already befriended two of the other older women. On top of that, because she didn't have her own car, her children arranged a transportation schedule so that she could see them and her grandchildren at least once a week. Her daughter beamed that my client was "like a new person." She seemed happy and no longer had crying spells out of the blue. She was motivated to wake up and get going every day. And she didn't have any complaints about her memory or attention! This client always sticks out in my mind as a prime example of the power of social engagement to improve mood and boost cognitive functioning.

## LET'S GET CONNECTED! PLANNING FOR YOUR SOCIALLY ACTIVE LIFE

Do you remember Amy, the student in one of my courses who committed to lifelong learning at the age of 73? Meet Ginger, Amy's classmate, a 57-year-old woman who is also working on her master's degree in gerontology. I gleaned from Ginger's comments in class that she was not only an active learner but also active outside of the classroom, so I asked her to share her story with us. She described an extensive social network that includes a large, close-knit family and a lot of friends. She stays socially connected by maintaining regular contact with her family and friends and participating in activities at her church. One of her hobbies, running with friends, combines physical and social elements. She explained that she and her friends counsel each other and try to solve problems in their lives during long runs. Ginger is a deacon at her church and serves on multiple church committees. She cotaught Sunday school to second- and third-grade children for more than 20 years, until the COVID pandemic hit. She is also a member of the Rebekah Circle, a group of church women, mostly in their 80s and 90s, who meet once a month for lunch and Bible study. She exclaimed that her "cognitive and spiritual life is enriched by friends from a wide spectrum of ages"!

Ginger gets doses of social connection by helping others. She described herself as "constantly scheming and brainstorming with family and church friends how to help someone get through a rough time or how to help celebrate someone's joy." For example, when her 96-year-old friend from church who has no family members around her moved into an assisted-living facility during the pandemic, Ginger helped her move and took on the responsibility of driving her to medical appointments. She also helps her church match people who are isolated and in need of human contact with parishioners who agree to call them regularly, and she makes flower arrangements and coordinates their deliveries to church members who need cheering up. What great ways to give back to the community while at the same time giving her brain a boost!

Without realizing it, Ginger is following many of the recommendations experts give for staying socially engaged. Experts on the Global Council on Brain Health came to a consensus about the best ways to maintain brain health through social engagement. In line with their recommendations, Ginger has a circle of friends and family with whom she can exchange ideas, thoughts, and concerns; she speaks with people in her network regularly; she helps others; she maintains social connections with people of different ages; and she is active in religious gatherings. She is also following the council's recommendation to maintain a variety of types of engagement. As we already learned about physical and cognitive activity, variety is the spice of life!

As with all brain-healthy behavior, social engagement is a lifelong process. It's important to build and maintain close relationships throughout our lives and to find ways to stay connected despite changes that might come with age or changes in life circumstances.

## Participate in Family, Cultural, and Community Events

Community and family events can provide fun and fulfilling opportunities to maintain social connections. From informal backyard barbecues to traditional cultural rituals and festivals, our families and communities are natural places to connect with other people. Share the cuisine, history, and art of your culture by attending culturally themed events with your family or in the community. Check your local newspaper or online media to learn about events around town, or plan your own event. Keep in mind that you can have a sense of community with whatever group of people you choose. For example, if family dynamics or distance make family gatherings an unappealing option, you might instead focus on social events within your religious group or with a circle of friends who have become like family to you. Share a meal, celebrate life events or holidays, or plan a group outing with your social circle, bringing people together based on your common bonds.

## Make It Meaningful

Have you heard of the term "generativity"? Coined by psychologist Erik Erikson, generativity is the desire to make a lasting contribution to the world. This desire tends to develop during middle age and generally involves a commitment to helping younger generations. Generativity can occur through different social roles at different points in life, such as raising children, volunteering, mentoring, or being a caregiver. Think about the Experience Corps Project discussed earlier. Senior volunteers share their wisdom from a lifetime of experiences with younger generations. This is a prime example of a social activity that fulfills a sense of generativity, which can provide a sense of purpose in life. Studies show that having a life purpose—seeing our lives as having meaning and a sense of direction, and having goals to live for—is associated with having a healthy brain. Why might that be? Scientists are not sure, but one possibility is that people who

| Add Meaning to Your Social Activities | | | |
|---|---|---|---|
| Focus on the relationships or social activities you enjoy the most | Turn to professionals who can assist if needed | Make a new connection or seek new opportunities to engage with others | If there are barriers to interacting with people, let someone assist you in making connections |
| Keep a circle of friends, family, or neighbors, & one or more confidants to communicate with routinely | If you are married, you should consider fostering other important relationships too | Try to communicate with your circle in person, or by phone, email, or other means | Help others, whether informally or through organizations or volunteer opportunities |
| Maintain social connections with people of different ages, including younger people | Add a new relationship or social activity you didn't try before | Be active and try groups, classes, or activities where you can meet and interact with others | If you are already socially active, diversify your activities |

*Note.* From "Engage Your Brain: GCBH Recommendations on Cognitively Stimulating Activities," July 2017 (https://www.aarp.org/content/dam/aarp/health/brain_health/2017/07/gcbh-cognitively-stimulating-activities-report-english-aarp.doi.10.26419%252Fpia.00001.001.pdf). Copyright 2017 by the Global Council on Brain Health. Adapted with permission.

feel like their life has meaning are more motivated to take care of their health. They are more likely to maintain health-promoting activities such as exercising, having a healthy diet, and keeping up with their medical care.

You can make your social activities more meaningful by giving or receiving support. One of Ginger's recommendations for staying socially engaged was "Seek a way to help others." Noting that so many organizations need help, such as reading to children or delivering meals to seniors, she added, "activities are especially rewarding when you know they're enriching other people's lives, and the people that you will get to know doing volunteer work are often some of the kindest and most interesting people you'll ever meet." You can do this through formal volunteerism or simply by providing social support to friends and family. Social support is any type of help that you give to other people or receive from other people. This can be emotional support (expressing empathy, love, trust, or caring), instrumental support (physical, tangible help, for example, providing transportation or meals for someone), or informational support (giving advice, suggestions, or information). Support goes both ways in meaningful relationships. Giving and receiving are both important. Think reciprocity.

## Be Flexible and Creative

The COVID pandemic forced us all to rethink how we maintain social connections. Physical distancing challenges our social lives in big and small ways, limiting our travel, preventing large gatherings, even causing us to question a handshake or hug that would have come naturally in the past. We are all learning—or trying to learn—to be flexible and creative in our social interactions. Even aside from COVID, though, different circumstances in life can challenge our ability to make connections to other people. Living in a rural area might limit your options for certain social activities due to having fewer people in your community and being physically isolated from others. Retirement can come with more isolation as you lose regular contact with colleagues during the work week. Relocating makes it necessary to find a new circle of local friends. Even becoming an empty nester can lead to feelings of loneliness when the usual contact with your children is gone. Regardless of our situation, to stay socially connected, we must remain flexible about finding options for social activity and try to be creative when circumstances limit us.

Many of us who lived before this era of digital technology went through a period of adjustment to get used to computer-based communication. I admit I wouldn't even consider using a social media platform for quite awhile, so I joined social media sites such as

Facebook and Instagram many years after most of my friends and family. Clearly, in-person contact is more ideal for most of us than email, text messages, social networking sites, or video calls. But research shows that digital social engagement still offers social rewards. For example, seniors who engage in online communities for older adults report feeling emotionally supported and intellectually stimulated. In general, internet use in older adults is linked to greater feelings of social connection and support, fewer feelings of loneliness and depression, and more positive attitudes about aging. Even if it requires a period of adjustment, consider expanding your social connections by taking advantage of the variety of options digital technology has to offer!

There are other ways to be creative as we plan for a socially engaged life. Did you know that the positive benefits of social connections extend to our interactions with our furry friends? Pet owners are less likely to report feelings of loneliness, especially if they feel a strong sense of attachment to their pets. One study surveyed adults 50 years and older, asking about whether they owned dogs and, if so, how frequently they walked their dogs. The respondents who walked their dogs at least four times per week reported a higher sense of community compared with people who didn't have a dog and the dog owners who took their pet on walks less frequently. This stronger sense of community might be due to dog walking serving as a catalyst for social interactions given that we typically encounter other people in our neighborhoods when we walk our dogs. Dogs can break the ice, triggering conversations and fostering a sense of community.

Regardless of the type of animal, taking care of a pet can give you a sense of purpose, which we know is an important element of social engagement. Studies show that interactions with animals have a range of physical and psychological benefits, including decreasing blood pressure, reducing symptoms of depression and anxiety, and reducing verbal aggression in people with Alzheimer's disease. Keeping in mind that not all studies find meaningful effects of interactions with animals on the body and the mind, it still seems worthwhile to consider owning a pet or spending time with animals in some other way. You might even try volunteering at an animal shelter to get multiple benefits—interactions with humans, interactions with animals, *and* a sense of purpose and meaning.

| **Let's Get Socially Connected!** | | |
|---|---|---|
| | Join or start a gardening club, book club, or arts and craft group | Audit a class at a local college |
| | Join a community sports team for adults or seniors | Join or start a walking, hiking, or bird watching group |
| | Take music lessons or join a choir or band | Get involved in a church, temple, or other religious organization |
| | Volunteer for a cause or group you're passionate about | Take group fitness or dance classes |
| | Play board games with friends or family | Write letters to a pen pal |
| | Cook or bake with someone else | Create a family tree or time capsule with family |
| | Check out local senior centers or meet-up groups | Join an organization, such as AARP, Red Hat Society, or SCORE |
| | Visit a local farmer's market | Participate in a local charity walk, and invite family and friends |
| | Join a theater group | Take a class related to a hobby |
| | Get on social media | Adopt a pet |
| | Become a mentor or tutor | Teach a class, such as an exercise, cooking, sewing, or dance class |

Digital technology and pet companionship are possible ways of overcoming social barriers of living in a rural environment, especially as broadband access is increasingly being expanded to rural communities. Still, staying socially connected in more isolated environments will require creativity and flexibility. Family, religious group, and volunteer activities can give you options. You can also consider taking the initiative yourself to form a social group centered on a shared hobby (e.g., a book club or adult sports league). And don't underestimate the connections you can maintain through activities as simple as making phone calls or having a pen pal! Check out the websites in the Resources and Suggested Readings section at the end of the chapter for more ideas.

## Tips for Success

You will get the most enjoyment and benefit from your social activity if you stay true to yourself and find ways to combine your social activities with other brain-healthy behavior, such as physical or cognitive activity.

### Be True to Yourself

Not everyone needs the same type or amount of social connection to be fulfilled, and that's OK! A conversation I had with one of my closest friends during the COVID pandemic comes to mind. As I lamented the challenges of being socially isolated because of the pandemic, she commented that for her, being able to stay home and interact less with people was the one silver lining to the situation. Rather than wanting regular contact with a large network of friends and acquaintances, as I do, she much prefers to have a limited circle of close friends and family and doesn't need or particularly want to interact with people outside that circle. Despite the differences in our social networks, we are both fulfilled and satisfied with the connections we have with other people under normal circumstances. On the other hand, someone in the throes of depression might have a strong urge to withdraw from other people, convinced that they will be better off if they shut everyone out. But in this case, social isolation actually makes them feel worse. It is best to intentionally reach out to friends and family when social withdrawal is due to depression rather than long-standing preferences based on your personality. We discuss depression and brain health in Chapter 7.

Our social preferences can also change with age. Laura Carstensen, professor of psychology at Stanford University, explains these changes with her *socioemotional selectivity theory*. This theory predicts that our time horizon shrinks as we age, so we prioritize emotionally meaningful goals and activities. When it comes to social engagement, this change in perspective leads many seniors to narrow their social networks so they can devote their emotional resources to fewer close friends and family. Studies have shown that people who choose to limit their social network in this way tend to be satisfied with their social connections. They report more positive social encounters and fewer negative encounters. This is another example of how the fulfillment we get from our social networks, and not necessarily the size of those networks, is most important to our health and happiness. When it comes to using social engagement as a tool to maintain a healthy brain, one size does not fit all. Our personality, culture, past relationships, and circumstances in life can all affect the type and amount of social connections we desire. Stay socially connected in the way that best suits you. Most important is that you seek social interactions that are pleasing and meaningful to you and that give you the benefits you want, whether that be enjoyment, support, a sense of purpose, or any other positive outcome that makes you feel connected with others.

## Combine Social Engagement With Physical or Cognitive Activity

To get the most brain-boosting bang for your buck, look for opportunities to combine social engagement with physical activity, cognitive activity, or both. As an example, you might find that working out with someone else motivates you to stick with your exercise plan, as we discussed in Chapter 2. This is exactly what happened to me when I first became physically active years ago. After a few years of sporadically exercising on my own, I finally became consistent when I started going to group exercise classes, which led to friendships with some of the regulars in the classes I attended. Not only did we spend time socializing before and after class, but we also started to plan group social events outside of class. We all looked forward to class for the social contact, which made us motivated to keep going. When I started teaching group fitness classes 10 years ago, I found that connecting with other people is the most rewarding part of being a fitness instructor. The classes I teach are all choreographed, so I have to stay mentally engaged to learn and teach the exercise routines. This means that teaching fitness class gives me a good dose of social, physical, and cognitive activity! Science tells us that the combination of social activity with exercise or cognitive engagement can give our brains a bigger boost than one type of activity alone. Try to incorporate activities into your life that involve multiple brain-healthy behaviors.

## SUMMARY

Remember these key points about staying socially engaged to maintain a healthy brain:

- People who are socially engaged—who interact with others, engage in purposeful activities with others, and maintain meaningful social relationships—tend to maintain their cognitive skills throughout life and may even be able to improve their cognitive functioning and reverse declines in the size of different parts of the brain.

- Social engagement promotes a sense of well-being and boosts mood, which can make it an effective treatment or prevention strategy for depression. This is not surprising because social engagement promotes the health of parts of the brain linked to depression.
- Social isolation can lead to loneliness. Loneliness is linked to cognitive decline and changes in the structure and function of the brain, including the buildup of brain markers for Alzheimer's disease.
- Increase your social connections by creating a circle of friends and family with whom you can exchange ideas, thoughts, and concerns, and interact with them regularly. Seek a variety of types of engagement, such as family and cultural events, religious activities, and volunteering.
- Make your social activities more meaningful by giving or receiving social support, but be true to yourself, knowing that not everyone desires the same type or amount of social connection.
- Remain flexible and try to be creative as you develop a socially active lifestyle. Consider making use of technology or interacting with animals in addition to in-person interactions with other people.
- Look for opportunities to engage in activities that combine social activity with exercise or a mental challenge, such as playing board games with family members or exercising with a friend.

## RESOURCES AND SUGGESTED READINGS

Global Council on Brain Health, "The Brain and Social Connectedness": https://www.aarp.org/content/dam/aarp/health/brain_health/2017/02/gcbh-social-engagement-report-english-aarp.doi.10.26419%252Fpia.00015.001.pdf

Science-based recommendations for staying socially connected to achieve a healthy brain.

**National Institute on Aging, "Participating in Activities You Enjoy":** https://www.nia.nih.gov/health/participating-activities-you-enjoy

Collection of ideas and resources to stay active as you age, many involving a social component. Includes a link to the website for Experience Corps, the program that matches volunteers 50 and older with schoolchildren who need tutoring in reading.

**AmeriCorps:** https://www.nationalservice.gov/

Government agency that connects with local partners to help you improve your local community through service projects and volunteerism. Includes AmeriCorps Seniors, formerly Senior Corps, which does the same for people aged 55 plus.

**engAGED: The National Resource Center for Engaging Older Adults:** https://www.engagingolderadults.org/

Designed to give professionals information about social engagement to share with their communities, but there are a lot of useful resources that anyone can use, including tips for staying socially engaged and links to the websites of other organizations addressing the social needs of older adults.

**Pets for the Elderly Foundation:** http://www.petsfortheelderly.org/

Organization that partners with local animal shelters to connect seniors with animals in need of a home. They help to pay adoption fees and provide pre-adoption veterinary care.

## SELECTED REFERENCES

Bzdok, D., & Dunbar, R. I. M. (2020). The neurobiology of social distance. *Trends in Cognitive Sciences*, *24*(9), 717–733. https://doi.org/10.1016/j.tics.2020.05.016

Cacioppo, S., Capitanio, J. P., & Cacioppo, J. T. (2014). Toward a neurology of loneliness. *Psychological Bulletin*, *140*(6), 1464–1504. https://doi.org/10.1037/a0037618

d'Oleire Uquillas, F., Jacobs, H. I. L., Biddle, K. D., Properzi, M., Hanseeuw, B., Schultz, A. P., Rentz, D. M., Johnson, K. A., Sperling, R. A., & Donovan, N. J. (2018). Regional tau pathology and loneliness in cognitively normal older adults. *Translational Psychiatry*, *8*(1), 282. https://doi.org/10.1038/s41398-018-0345-x

Donovan, N. J., Wu, Q., Rentz, D. M., Sperling, R. A., Marshall, G. A., & Glymour, M. M. (2017). Loneliness, depression and cognitive function in older U.S. adults. *International Journal of Geriatric Psychiatry*, *32*(5), 564–573. https://doi.org/10.1002/gps.4495

Gee, N. R., Mueller, M. K., & Curl, A. L. (2017). Human–animal interaction and older adults: An overview. *Frontiers in Psychology*, *8*, 1416. https://doi.org/10.3389/fpsyg.2017.01416

Guiney, H., Keall, M., & Machado, L. (2021). Volunteering in older adulthood is associated with activity engagement and cognitive functioning. *Aging, Neuropsychology, and Cognition*, *28*(2), 253–269. https://doi.org/10.1080/13825585.2020.1743230

Hajek, A., Brettschneider, C., Mallon, T., Ernst, A., Mamone, S., Wiese, B., Weyerer, S., Werle, J., Pentzek, M., Fuchs, A., Stein, J., Luck, T., Bickel, H., Weeg, D., Wagner, M., Heser, K., Maier, W., Scherer, M. Riedel-Heller, S. G., & König, H.-H. (2017). The impact of social engagement on health-related quality of life and depressive symptoms in old age—Evidence from a multicenter prospective cohort study in Germany. *Health and Quality of Life Outcomes*, *15*(1), 140. https://doi.org/10.1186/s12955-017-0715-8

Harada, K., Masumoto, K., & Kondo, N. (2019). Exercising alone or exercising with others and mental health among middle-aged and older adults: Longitudinal analysis of cross-lagged and simultaneous effects. *Journal of Physical Activity and Health*, *16*(7), 556–564. https://doi.org/10.1123/jpah.2018-0366

Kelly, M. E., Duff, H., Kelly, S., McHugh Power, J. E., Brennan, S., Lawlor, B. A., & Loughrey, D. G. (2017). The impact of social activities, social networks, social support and social relationships on the cognitive functioning of healthy older adults: A systematic review. *Systematic Reviews*, *6*(1), 259. https://doi.org/10.1186/s13643-017-0632-2

Kuiper, J. S., Zuidersma, M., Zuidema, S. U., Burgerhof, J. G., Stolk, R. P., Oude Voshaar, R. C., & Smidt, N. (2016). Social relationships and cognitive decline: A systematic review and meta-analysis of longitudinal cohort studies. *International Journal of Epidemiology, 45*(4), 1169–1206. https://doi.org/10.1093/ije/dyw089

Levasseur, M., Routhier, S., Clapperton, I., Dore, C., & Gallagher, F. (2020). Social participation needs of older adults living in a rural regional county municipality: Toward reducing situations of isolation and vulnerability. *BMC Geriatrics, 20*(1), 456. https://doi.org/10.1186/s12877-020-01849-5

Lewis, N. A., & Hill, P. L. (2020). Does being active mean being purposeful in older adulthood? Examining the moderating role of retirement. *Psychology and Aging, 35*(7), 1050–1057. https://doi.org/10.1037/pag0000568

Lutz, J., Van Orden, K. A., Bruce, M. L., & Conwell, Y. (2021). Social disconnection in late life suicide: An NIMH workshop on state of the research in identifying mechanisms, treatment targets, and interventions. *American Journal of Geriatric Psychiatry.* Advance online publication. https://doi.org/10.1016/j.jagp.2021.01.137

Moored, K. D., Chan, T., Varma, V. R., Chuang, Y. F., Parisi, J. M., & Carlson, M. C. (2020). Engagement in enriching early-life activities is associated with larger hippocampal and amygdala volumes in community-dwelling older adults. *Journals of Gerontology: Series B. Psychological Sciences and Social Sciences, 75*(8), 1637–1647. https://doi.org/10.1093/geronb/gby150

Mwilambwe-Tshilobo, L., Ge, T., Chong, M., Ferguson, M. A., Misic, B., Burrow, A. L., Leahy, R. M., & Spreng, R. N. (2019). Loneliness and meaning in life are reflected in the intrinsic network architecture of the brain. *Social Cognitive and Affective Neuroscience, 14*(4), 423–433. https://doi.org/10.1093/scan/nsz021

Sharifian, N., Zaheed, A. B., Morris, E. P., Sol, K., Manly, J. J., Schupf, N., Mayeux, R., Brickman, A. M., & Zahodne, L. B. (2021). Social network characteristics moderate associations between cortical thickness and cognitive functioning in older adults. *Alzheimer's and Dementia.* Advance online publication. https://doi.org/10.1002/alz.12383

Wilson, R. S., Krueger, K. R., Arnold, S. E., Schneider, J. A., Kelly, J. F., Barnes, L. L., Tang, Y., & Bennett, D. A. (2007). Loneliness and risk of

Alzheimer disease. *Archives of General Psychiatry*, 64(2), 234–240. https://doi.org/10.1001/archpsyc.64.2.234

Zhou, Z., Wang, P., & Fang, Y. (2018). Social engagement and its change are associated with dementia risk among Chinese older adults: A longitudinal study. *Scientific Reports*, 8(1), 1551. https://doi.org/10.1038/s41598-017-17879-w

CHAPTER 5

# YOU ARE WHAT YOU EAT: NUTRITION FOR A HEALTHY BRAIN

Sometimes in life, we build up so much expectation about an event or experience that, once it actually happens, we feel let down. That was not at all what happened when I traveled to Greece! The anticipation was high beforehand, but somehow the trip exceeded my expectations in every way. The history, the architecture, the breathtaking scenery—all of it filled me with awe and amazement. But what I think I enjoyed the most was the food. My favorite was the seafood, served mere hours after being caught. I will never forget sitting on the patio at a restaurant in the Athens marina, marveling when the server brought to the table a basket of whole, fresh fish that had just been caught and invited my travel companions and me to choose which fish we wanted and how we wanted it to be cooked. You can't get much fresher than that! I couldn't have enough of the succulent fruits and vegetables—I swear the tomatoes were the juiciest, sweetest tomatoes I've ever had! And the olive oil made me wonder what I had been calling "olive oil" all my life. Since that trip, I have been trying to find the closest possible approximations to the cuisine I savored in Greece. I even took a cooking class in Greece so that I could continue making some of my favorite dishes at home, like spinach pie, dolmades, and moussaka. And that's great news for my brain health! The Mediterranean diet, which is filled with vegetables, fruits, fish, whole grains, and extra virgin olive oil, has a number of health benefits, including promoting a healthy brain. Much of what we know about this comes from what nutrition science has told us about vitamins, minerals, and micronutrients.

In this chapter, we will delve into what research does—and does not—tell us about how our diets affect our brains. We will do some myth-busting about supplements that claim to boost brain power or prevent dementia. You will get practical guidance on how to establish better dietary habits, taking small steps until you reach your goal.

## WHAT RESEARCH TELLS US

You have probably experienced the same "nutrition whiplash" that I have. One day, you see a news headline that touts the benefits of some food or ingredient, followed a few months or even weeks later by a headline that claims the same food is bad for you. The example I always think of is the decades-long debate over eggs. Part of the challenge is that modern nutrition science is relatively young, dating back only to the 1920s, when the first vitamin was isolated. For a few decades after that, nutrition researchers focused on *micronutrients*: vitamins and minerals, such as iron and Vitamin D, that are needed only in small amounts but are still important for optimal health. They must be derived from our diet because our bodies do not produce them.

The emphasis on particular vitamins and minerals started a trend of focusing on linking single nutrients to specific diseases. Take, for example, fat and sugar, both of which have been vilified for years as the cause of obesity, cardiovascular disease, and other illnesses. The problem with this reductionist approach is that it is too simple. Over time, advances in nutrition science have shown that the combination of different nutrients in our diets influences our health. Diet *patterns*, not just specific nutrients, are most important for health and wellness. And this is true for maintaining a healthy brain.

**What's Good for Your Heart Is Good for Your Brain**

In my clinical practice, the vast majority of my clients have one or more risk factors for heart disease—conditions such as high blood pressure, high cholesterol, or diabetes, all of which make them vulnerable to heart attack or stroke. This is not surprising given that I specialize in the neuropsychological assessment of older adults, and these types of medical conditions become more common the older we get. It's also not surprising because clients come to see me with concerns about their memory and cognitive skills, and diseases that affect our heart are among the most common causes of cognitive decline as we age. This is because the health of our heart's blood vessels directly influences the health of our brain's blood vessels, as we discuss in Chapter 7. When it comes to nutrition, what this means is that a diet that benefits your heart also benefits your brain. But what dietary patterns are best for your heart?

The diet most consistently linked to good heart health—and brain health—is the Mediterranean-style diet, common in countries bordering the Mediterranean Sea such as Greece, Italy, and Spain. To be clear, there is not *one* diet across these disparate countries; instead, they all have common characteristics that benefit our hearts and our brains:

- Lots of vegetables, fruits, whole grains, potatoes, beans, and healthy fats, such as monounsaturated and polyunsaturated fats, which are found in some types of nuts, seeds, and fish, among other foods. Olive oil is typically the primary fat source for preparing food.
- Moderate amounts of eggs, dairy products, and poultry.
- Limited red meat, refined grains, and sweets.
- Moderate amounts of wine.

Study after study has demonstrated the health benefits of this type of diet. It can lower the risk of cardiovascular disease and stroke, help manage diabetes, and protect against cognitive decline as we age. The Mediterranean-style diet has even been linked to a longer life span!

Another heart-healthy diet is DASH (Dietary Approaches to Stop Hypertension), which emphasizes low sodium intake and small portion sizes in addition to many of the components of the Mediterranean-style diet, such as an emphasis on fruits, vegetables, nuts, lean meats, fish, whole grains, and heart healthy fats. Studies have shown that DASH lowers blood pressure and can help prevent osteoporosis, cancer, heart disease, stroke, and diabetes.

A few years ago, researchers at Rush University in Chicago created a new diet called the Mediterranean–DASH Intervention for Neurodegenerative Delay (MIND) diet. This diet was specifically designed to promote brain health. As the name implies, the MIND diet combines elements of the Mediterranean and DASH diets, in particular the emphasis on vegetables, nuts, beans, whole grains, poultry, and fish. The MIND diet also recommends different food groups on the basis of their potential benefits to brain health, including leafy green vegetables and blueberries, and food groups that should be limited because of their potential to have negative effects on brain health, including red meat, butter and stick margarine, cheese, pastries and sweets, and fried or fast food. Because this diet is fairly new, there are only a few research studies to speak to its impact on our brains. But there is already evidence that older adults who stick to this diet show less cognitive decline over a nearly 5-year period and can delay the onset of Alzheimer's disease.

Although all of this seems to make clear that a heart-healthy diet is a brain-healthy diet, we should note a few caveats to dietary research. Because it's not feasible to completely control human diets for extended periods of time, research that links dietary patterns to health by and large must rely on the reports that research volunteers make of what they eat and drink. The researchers then look for patterns between dietary habits and health outcomes such as high blood pressure, obesity, memory loss, or dementia. This can certainly give us a clue about links between nutrition and the brain, but we have to remember that these links do not necessarily mean that the dietary patterns directly caused the improvements in brain health. It could be, for example, that the people who closely follow the diet are more likely to exercise regularly or have strong family support and that these characteristics give the brain a boost. And, of course, it is also possible that people are not completely honest when they report what they eat and drink. But even with these caveats in mind, the sheer number of studies that point in the same direction— that heart health equals brain health—is enough for me to advise my clients to keep a heart-healthy diet, and to do the same myself!

## Typical Western Diets Are Not Good for Your Brain

Keeping in mind that our overall dietary pattern is what's most important, scientific studies do show us that certain parts of our diet increase our risk for heart disease, which in turn can impact our brain. For example, research suggests possible health problems linked to staples of what is considered the typical Western diet, a high-calorie diet that includes high intake of red meat, sugar, saturated fat, salt, and refined grains.

One example comes from trans fats, the "partially hydrogenated oils" found in many processed foods, such as frozen pizza, margarines, and fried foods. Trans fats raise your levels of low-density lipoprotein cholesterol, often called the "bad" cholesterol, and lower your levels of high-density lipoprotein cholesterol, considered the "good" cholesterol. People who have a diet high in trans fat have a higher risk of heart disease, stroke, and Type 2 diabetes compared with people with less trans fat in their diet. Research shows that trans fats can permeate brain cells, altering the communication between them. This can lead to problems such as cognitive impairment and depression.

Again, it is most likely the combination of certain types of food, especially in large amounts, that spells trouble for our brains. Your best bet for maintaining a healthy brain through nutrition is to develop long-term healthy eating habits based on foods most consistently linked to a healthy heart—such as fruits, vegetables, whole grains, lean meats and fish, beans, and nuts—and to limit your intake of trans fats, salt, and added sugars.

## FOOD GUIDELINES

**EAT REGULARLY**

Berries
Fresh vegetables, especially leafy greens
Healthy fats (such as extra virgin olive oil)
A moderate amount of nuts
Fish and other seafood

. . . . . . . . . . . . . . . . . . . . . . . . . . . . . . . .

**INCLUDE**

Beans and other legumes
Fruits (in addition to berries)
Low fat dairy, such as yogurt
Poultry
Grains

. . . . . . . . . . . . . . . . . . . . . . . . . . . . . . . .

**LIMIT**

Fried food
Pastries
Processed foods
Red meat
Red meat products
Whole fat dairy, such as cheese and butter
Salt

*Note.* From "Brain Food: GCBH Recommendations on Nourishing Your Brain Health," January 2018 (https://www.aarp.org/content/dam/aarp/health/brain_health/2018/01/gcbh-recommendations-on-nourishing-your-brain-health.doi.10.26419%252Fpia.00019.001.pdf). Copyright 2018 by the Global Council on Brain Health. Adapted with permission.

## Supplements Are Not All They're Cracked Up to Be

According to a 2019 survey by the AARP, 81% of Americans age 50 and older believe supplements are important for overall health, and over one quarter regularly take supplements for their brain health. As a proponent of the power of healthy behavior to build healthy brains, I am disheartened when I think about these numbers. I'm not going to mince words here: Dietary supplements for brain health are a waste of money. Now that I've already cut to the chase, let's back up and talk about why I have this professional opinion, a conclusion that is shared by experts from the Global Council on Brain Health.

As a perfect example of the concerns about supplements, consider the case of Prevagen. Prevagen made millions of dollars more than $165 million from 2007 to 2015, according to the Federal Trade Commission—by making unsubstantiated claims that their supplement was the answer to the memory and cognitive concerns of older adults. The company had ads everywhere, including NBC, Fox News, CNN—you name it. No wonder they were able to dupe so many people! A Federal Trade Commission report concluded: "The marketers of Prevagen preyed on the fears of older consumers experiencing age-related memory loss. But one critical thing these marketers forgot is that their claims need to be backed up by real scientific evidence."

According to multiple reports, including one from Harvard University, the main ingredient in Prevagen is a dietary protein called *apoaequorin*, which was first discovered in glowing jellyfish. There is no evidence that apoaequorin has a role in human memory; also, experts doubt that ingesting it could ultimately affect the brain. But the marketers capitalized on a small subset of people in their research studies whose memory scores slightly improved after taking the supplement to make wide-sweeping claims about the power of

Prevagen. As I worked on this chapter, I found it disturbing that because this case remains in litigation the company was still in business. And their website continues to claim that their product "has been clinically shown to help with mild memory loss associated with aging," albeit with fine print at the bottom of the page: "These statements have not been evaluated by the Food and Drug Administration. This product is not intended to diagnose, treat, cure or prevent any disease."

Prevagen is a prime example of the problem with dietary supplements, but it is only one of the estimated 50,000 supplements that claim to improve mood, brain function, and overall health with little or no evidence. In 2015, a meta-analysis combining the results of 24 different studies on brain health supplements concluded that supplements had no impact on cognitive functioning in middle-age and older adults.

Even worse, not only are supplements ineffective, they can be downright unsafe! That's because the U.S. Food and Drug Administration does not require the same level of review and approval of supplements as they do for food products and drugs. As a result, you never know what you're getting when you pick out a supplement in a store or online. The quality, content, purity, and potency vary from product to product. Potential toxicity varies, too. In fact, a September 2020 article on the *Consumer Reports* website warned, "A new analysis found high levels of potentially dangerous pharmaceuticals in some supplements available in the U.S." This warning was based on the results of a study that evaluated the content of 10 supplements that claimed to boost memory. The team of researchers found that most of the supplement labels listed inaccurate quantities of important ingredients. This issue is so important, in fact, that other countries require a prescription for many of them. On top of that, some of the supplements included unapproved drugs that were not even listed on their labels! Some of the ingredients that were inaccurately listed or not listed at all have been associated with serious side effects and complications, such as sedation, blood pressure changes, insomnia, agitation, dependence, and hospitalization.

Supplements are not a good choice for building and maintaining a healthy brain. This is not to say that the vitamins and minerals in some supplements are unimportant. Actually, there *is* evidence that nutrients such as omega-3 fatty acids and Vitamin D play an important role in health. But experts advise that most people will get enough of these vitamins from food if they follow a healthy, varied diet. Unless your doctor has told you that you have a specific nutritional deficiency, then diet, not taking supplements, is the best way to get important nutrients.

## NOURISH YOUR BRAIN! DEVELOPING HEALTHY EATING HABITS FOR A HEALTHY BRAIN

We can benefit from a healthy diet at any age but, like all brain-boosting behavior, the sooner you start, the better. But what is the best way to start and maintain healthy eating habits? And how can we overcome the barriers that threaten our success? I posed these and other questions about nutrition to Julia Kelly, a registered dietitian who provides medical nutrition therapy and nutrition counseling in different corporate settings and for clients in my brain health company, CerebroFit.

In Julia's experience, relying on healthy eating "solutions" from others creates roadblocks when we try to start and maintain healthy eating habits. We often hear stories about "one habit" or "this diet" that led to dramatic weight loss or other health benefits and assume we will get the same results. According to Julia, though, "This often leads people down a path of dietary changes that have limited bearing on the challenges they face in their day-to-day life." She pointed out that we all have individual challenges and goals, so what works for someone else might not work for you. "People often need to spend a little time with themselves rather than sifting through all the different diets and tricks they are bombarded with," she advised. "It is critical that those trying to change eating habits take some time to reflect on where their individual eating problems lie so they can find the right solution for them."

The "individual eating problems" Julia mentioned include our personal histories, eating habits, and relationship to food, all of which can create barriers to success. Examples include the challenge of learning how to reduce or replace foods in your diet that you have eaten since childhood. The solution may be to explore new foods or learn to cook the same dishes in healthier ways. Another hurdle might be a lack of consistent eating patterns and rushing through meals. Positive changes in this case may be to wake up 15 minutes earlier in the day to eat breakfast or blocking time in your workday for lunch. Other people might struggle with emotional eating; over-eating; or difficulty preparing quick, low-cost meals. As Julia told me, "Each of these barriers, and their solutions, are really different. Cookie cutter eating plans focus heavily on addressing physical hunger and are really inadequate to handle psychological eating cues." Psychological eating cues can range from stress, to slack of sleep, to relationship problems. Often, it's our response to these cues that drive our unhealthy eating, even more so than our food selection or portion sizes. Whether you work with a nutrition professional like Julia or on your own, a self-assessment of your eating habits will help you identify your barriers to developing healthier eating habits.

### Consider Journaling

Julia recommends that you assess your eating habits before trying to decide on a course of action. You can do this by spending a few days or a few weeks noting your eating habits in a journal without trying to make changes yet. Julia emphasized that this step should be done *without judgment.* What should you include in this journal?

First, take stock of your current eating habits. You want to address some of these questions:

- What did you eat?
- How hungry where you prior to your meals? How full were you after?
- When, where, and why did you eat?
- How many times did you eat?
- Were you doing anything else while you ate?
- How were you feeling before your meal? As you ate? After your meal?
- Where did the food come from? Who prepared it?
- If you didn't prepare it, why not?

Next, think about your history of eating habits. Consider these questions:

- Was there a period of time when your weight (or substitute any other health metric) increased?
- Was this a short period of time, or gradual?
- What else was going on during this time?
- What habits changed during this time?
- What special diets have you followed in the past? What did you like or dislike about them?
- When was the last time you felt healthy and happy with your eating habits?
- What habits are the most challenging to maintain?

Once you've considered your history, think ahead to the future. Write down what success looks like to you, remembering that this can be different for all of us. This chapter focuses on establishing healthy eating habits for a healthier brain, but you might have other long-term goals you hope to achieve, such as losing weight, getting your blood sugar under control, or improving other aspects of your health. In your journal, answer these questions:

- What do health and healthy eating mean to you? What does healthy eating do for you?
- What are some eating habits and routines you would like to have in place in 1 year or 5 years?
- What resources do you need to support your success?

Julia deems the next step as the most important: Review the habits you wrote down in your journal. She explained,

> The benefit that comes from journaling is not monitoring your decision making at every meal so you make the healthiest possible decision every time you eat. It is really taking the time to reflect on and analyze the events and thoughts that are driving eating habits. (J. Kelly, personal communication, October 29, 2020)

Go through your journal and note key takeaways. You may have only one or two, or you may have many. Either way, this is valuable information to help you plan for healthy eating. Here are some questions to help you identify valuable nuggets of information from your eating journal:

- Do you feel meal consistency (*when* you eat) or meal composition (*what* you eat) is the bigger challenge? Are weekdays or weekends more challenging?
- How do mood, stress, environments, or relationships drive your eating habits?

- In what ways do your current habits align or misalign with your definitions of success?

The next step is to prioritize. Pick two or three of your takeaways to focus on, in particular, ones that align with your own definition of success around healthy eating. Then you can set actionable, realistic goals—goals that allow you to plan clear, attainable steps. You can also use this journaling exercise to identify sources of support for your healthy eating journey, such as cooking lessons or counseling for learning to manage your emotions.

## Think Balance

I cringe when I hear the term "superfood," which seems to be a mainstay in magazines, news stories, and marketing material for foods and beverages. The idea of a superfood comes from marketers who found a catchy way of describing foods—such as blueberries, kale, and acai—that are thought to be good for health because they are packed with nutrients. While many of the so-called superfoods do in fact contain nutrients that benefit health, my objection to the term stems from the fact that there is no official definition for a superfood from any scientific or regulatory agency. This means that what gets labeled as a superfood can be arbitrary, based more on marketing and less on science. Also, the labeling can give the inaccurate impression that eating one or more of the superfoods is all we need to be healthy.

But when it comes to nutrition for brain health, there is no silver bullet. Benefit comes from dietary patterns that include a balanced combination of different types of food that contain different types of nutrients. So, rather than eating blueberries three times a day because you read a story about how nutritious they are, incorporate into your meal plan a variety of nutritious berries, vegetables, whole grains, and the other foods we discussed that have been linked to better health.

## Consider Your Age and Health Needs

Even though there are general nutrition principles for a healthy brain, one size does not fit all. Depending on your age, medical conditions, and other special circumstances, you might have specific nutritional needs. For example, as we age, we are more vulnerable to deficiencies in vitamins B12, B6, and riboflavin. Research suggests this is due to a combination of getting less of the B vitamins in our diet, our bodies absorbing less of the vitamins from our food, and the body needing more of these particular vitamins to maintain health in our

| Practical Tips for Healthy Eating | | | |
|---|---|---|---|
| Stay physically active to complement eating a healthy diet | Avoid eating in excess | Eat at least one meal per week with fish that is not fried | Look at the sodium content in prepared foods you are eating |
| Use vinegar, lemon, aromatic herbs, and spices to increase flavor in food without increasing salt | Consider dietary counseling if you are trying to overcome medical conditions | Snack on raw, plain, unsalted nuts; they may be beneficial for brain health | Eat a wide variety of different colored vegetables |
| Choose fresh, frozen, or canned fruits and vegetables stored in water or their own juice | Purchase food and prepare meals at home | Use mono and polyunsaturated fats in cooking | Read packaged food labels to help you choose healthier options |

*Note.* From "Brain Food: GCBH Recommendations on Nourishing Your Brain Health," January 2018 (https://www.aarp.org/content/dam/aarp/health/brain_health/2018/01/gcbh-recommendations-on-nourishing-your-brain-health.doi.10.26419%252Fpia.00019.001.pdf). Copyright 2018 by the Global Council on Brain Health. Adapted with permission.

senior years. Lack of B vitamins has been linked to cardiovascular disorders, which can in turn affect our brains. Because of the susceptibility to vitamin B deficiency, older adults might require a diet full of more poultry, dairy products, dark leafy greens, and other foods rich in vitamin B. Many chronic medical conditions, such as diabetes, also require dietary changes for optimal health. As you grow older, or if you receive a new medical diagnosis, it is wise to talk to your physician to find out if you should make any changes to your dietary habits. In some situations it might be helpful to see a dietitian such as Julia, a food and nutrition expert who provides medical nutrition therapy and nutritional counseling that are backed by science and tailored to meet each person's needs.

## Tips for Success

In your journey to healthier eating habits, take small steps toward your ultimate goal, avoid making last-minute decisions about your meals, and find ways to make healthy eating enjoyable.

### Take It One Step at a Time

Most of us have been in the same boat at some time in our lives: We start a diet as a New Year's resolution, or we want to lose weight before a wedding or big vacation, so we make drastic changes to our eating habits in the hope of getting dramatic results. But usually we stick to our new diet for a few weeks, at best, before returning to old habits. And even if we do lose any weight during our brief foray into healthier eating, we most likely regain those lost pounds. It is tough to change our diets! It takes time, effort, sometimes money, and a lot of organization. And it can be incredibly frustrating and demoralizing to keep trying to make long-term changes without success.

The goal is to develop a lifelong dietary pattern that is good for your brain as well as the rest of your body. Instead of trying to overhaul your diet and setting yourself up for disappointment, make small changes that you can then build on. This is a marathon, not a sprint, so take it one step at a time. Small changes can go a long way. For example, according to a 2017 article in the *Journal of the American Medical Association*, increasing fruit intake by just one serving each day can reduce the chance of death due to cardiovascular disease by 8%. That's the equivalent of 60,000 fewer deaths annually in the United States! The same article recommended small steps, such as reducing consumption of sugar-sweetened beverages, fast food, processed meats, and sweets, while increasing vegetables, legumes (or beans), nuts, and whole grains. Notice that these recommendations are similar to guidelines from the Mediterranean-style diet.

Julia encourages her clients to start conservatively and focus on making those small changes consistent. Remember that you can prioritize two or three takeaway points from your food journal as a start. Also, remember that life happens, so inevitably you will have times when even those small changes are difficult to maintain. Don't get discouraged in these situations! Instead, you can intentionally pull back temporarily, limiting your focus on one or two habits in the short term, and then go back to pursuing your larger, long-term goals when the time is right.

Take it one step at a time, but keep your long-term goals in mind. This is especially true when we think about eating to promote a healthy brain, because we can't monitor success in the same way that we can monitor weight or blood sugar levels. And even some of the more measurable health goals, such as weight loss, can take time to achieve. To keep your motivation over the long haul, focus on a lifestyle change instead of a quick fix for a short-term goal.

PLAN AHEAD

Good nutrition requires planning. It takes planning to make sure that you get enough of the nutrients that are good for your brain, and it takes planning to avoid making last-minute decisions about food. Last-minute food choices typically include less healthy food, such as fast food and processed food, out of convenience or necessity. As we discussed for exercise, cognitive activity, and social activity, the best way to make lifestyle changes is to plan for them.

I find it useful to plan my meals and snacks for the week before I shop for groceries. I try to incorporate nutrition guidelines when

- Plan when you are going to eat and block this time into your schedule.

- Consider no-cook breakfast and lunch options that are fully prepared.

- Make cooking more efficient. For example, on the weekends, prep items that take a while to cook and store them in the fridge or freezer until they will be used.

- Plan meals that can be eaten over multiple days. Crock-Pot, sheet pan, or one pot meals often can be cooked in large portions using minimal dishes.

- Keep meals simple. It can reduce the level of prep work involved and the amount of dishes used in the process.

- Clean as you go. Dishes are often much easier to wash right after they were used.

- Prep meals that can be eaten over a series of days and buy your meal components in bulk.

- Plan meals in advance to reduce food waste and impulse buying at the grocery store. Keep meals simple to avoid stocking up on unique ingredients that only get used once.

- Eat out less, and when you do eat out, consider splitting your meal with someone else or taking home leftovers for another meal.

- Use benefits from government programs such as SNAP and WIC if you're eligible.

- Replace meat and seafood with dried legumes and whole grains, inexpensive alternatives that can be prepped in bulk and frozen for later use.

- Shop smarter. Reduce unwholesome snack foods and expensive convenience items, such as cut up or peeled produce. Stick with store brands. Prioritize food in season, which is often on sale. Peruse coupons and join your supermarket's shoppers club.

**Overcoming Barriers of Time and Money**

I make my food schedule. For example, I include berries and leafy greens in my meals and snacks for the week, and I try to have fish once a week. I have a document that I update weekly with my plans for breakfast, lunch, dinner, and snacks for each day of the week. As an aside, I actually include my exercise plans for each day in the same document, as a way of making sure I'm balancing out cardiovascular exercise, strength training, and yoga across my week. I then make my grocery list, and I incorporate the guidelines when I shop, such as opting for fresh fruits and vegetables over canned ones. This is just one example of how you might plan ahead for a healthy diet. Another option is to plan a month-long menu of easy meals for breakfast, lunch, and dinner. This can help reduce the time you spend each week organizing food for the following week. Plus, it can be reused or slightly modified as needed throughout the year. There are a variety of websites and apps that some people find helpful for making a healthy eating plan, some of which are provided at the end of this chapter. See what works for you.

## Make It Enjoyable

Have you noticed that when a character on a TV show or movie tries to lose weight, they seem to only eat bland food, like dry salads or rice cakes? This extreme behavior might make for a comical storyline, but it paints a negative—and inaccurate—picture about healthy eating. You can have healthy eating habits and truly enjoy food! Variety in your diet is a good thing, so there is no need to limit yourself to just a few foods or types of food. If you start a diet that is too restrictive, you will be less likely to enjoy your meals and thus less likely to stick to it. As Julia pointed out, restrictive diets

> can create feelings of guilt or shame when the person following this diet is unable to stay on plan. And they can lead to cycles of extreme restriction and binging in response to feelings of deprivation or frustration. Over time, this can take a physical

and psychological toll that is really hard to break out of, particularly if these habits have been a part of someone's life for many years. (J. Kelly, personal communication, October 29, 2020)

Restrictive diets are often socially isolating. Because lifestyle changes are usually difficult, wide ranging, and time consuming, it's important that the journey be more enjoyable than isolating. Julia advises her clients to start by focusing on changes in their eating habits that they find somewhat enjoyable and to enlist support for their healthy eating journey that offers motivation and accountability. Support can include friends, family, or professional help as well as podcasts, books, and social media pages that drive positive self-talk. She also encourages clients to put time into experimenting, whether that is trying new foods, new cooking strategies, or new exercise options, which go hand in hand with healthy eating.

Add enjoyment to your healthy eating journey by combining it with other brain-healthy behavior, such as social engagement or cognitive engagement. Take a cooking class with a friend. Plan fun cooking activities for the family at home. This is a great time to teach cooking skills to kids! Learn a new cooking technique that provides a mental challenge. Try gardening as a way of getting physical activity and growing healthy vegetables and herbs at the same time. Think outside of the box, but one way or the other, try to make healthy eating fun instead of a chore!

## SUMMARY

Remember these key points about healthy eating to maintain a healthy brain:

- To maintain a healthy brain, develop long-term healthy eating habits that include a balanced combination of various types of food and different types of nutrients.

- What's good for your heart is good for your brain! Heart-healthy diets, such as the Mediterranean-style diet, DASH, and the MIND diet, are great options. They all emphasize fruits, vegetables, whole grains, lean meats and fish, beans, and nuts.
- The traditional Western diet is high in calories and includes a high intake of red meat, sugar, saturated fat, salt, and refined grains. This dietary pattern is linked to heart problems and other diseases, so limit your intake of those types of food.
- Dietary supplements are usually ineffective, and they can even be unsafe. It's best to get your nutrients from eating a balanced diet, unless your doctor tells you that you have a specific nutritional deficiency that requires supplementation.
- To develop healthy eating habits, think about your personal challenges, goals, eating habits, and history. What works for someone else might not work for you. Consider journaling to gain insight into your eating habits, and develop personal goals that make sense for you.
- Don't try to overhaul your diet; instead, make small changes that you can build on.
- Plan ahead for your meals to avoid making last-minute decisions about food, which are usually less healthy decisions.
- Enjoy your food! Don't make your diet overly restrictive. Add enjoyment by keeping your meals varied, learning new recipes, or adding a social element.

## RESOURCES AND SUGGESTED READINGS

**Global Council on Brain Health, "Brain Food":** https://www.aarp.org/content/dam/aarp/health/brain_health/2018/01/gcbh-recommendations-on-nourishing-your-brain-health.doi.10.26419%252Fpia.00019.001.pdf
More information about nutrition and brain health from an international group of brain experts.

**Global Council on Brain Health, "The Real Deal on Brain Health Supplements":** https://www.aarp.org/content/dam/aarp/health/brain_health/2019/06/gcbh-supplements-report-english.doi.10.26419-2Fpia.00094.001.pdf

Summary of what scientists know and what we still need to learn about supplements and brain health.

**U.S. Department of Agriculture, "My Plate":** https://www.choosemyplate.gov/

Information and resources to help you plan and stick to a healthy diet, including a link to the MyPlate app, which lets you pick daily food goals, track your progress, and join challenges with other people. Includes healthy recipes, too!

**National Institute on Aging, "Healthy Eating":** https://www.nia.nih.gov/health/healthy-eating

Great collection of news stories and other articles about nutrition and health, including tips for eating healthy on a budget and overcoming roadblocks to healthy eating.

**American Heart Association, "Healthy Living":** https://www.heart.org/en/healthy-living

Lots of resources to help you eat smart and lose weight. Also includes information and tools for other healthy behaviors you're learning about in this book, including exercise, sleep, and keeping a healthy heart.

## SELECTED REFERENCES

Amini, Y., Saif, N., Greer, C., Hristov, H., & Isaacson, R. (2020). The role of nutrition in individualized Alzheimer's risk reduction. *Current Nutrition Reports, 9*(2), 55–63. https://doi.org/10.1007/s13668-020-00311-7

Ballarini, T., Melo van Lent, D., Brunner, J., Schroder, A., Wolfsgruber, S., Altenstein, S., Brosseron, F., Buerger, K., Dechent, P., Dobisch, L.,

Düzel, E., Ertl-Wagner, B., Fliessbach, K., Freiesleben, S. D., Frommann, I., Glanz, W., Hauser, D., Haynes, J. D., Heneka, M. T., . . . Wagner, M. (2021). Mediterranean diet, Alzheimer disease biomarkers and brain atrophy in old age. *Neurology, 96*(24). Advance online publication. https://doi.org/10.1212/WNL.0000000000012067

Crawford, C., Boyd, C., Avula, B., Wang, Y. H., Khan, I. A., & Deuster, P. A. (2020). A public health issue: Dietary supplements promoted for brain health and cognitive performance. *The Journal of Alternative and Complementary Medicine, 26*(4), 265–272. https://doi.org/10.1089/acm.2019.0447

de Ridder, D., Kroese, F., Evers, C., Adriaanse, M., & Gillebaart, M. (2017). Healthy diet: Health impact, prevalence, correlates, and interventions. *Psychology & Health, 32*(8), 907–941. https://doi.org/10.1080/08870446.2017.1316849

Ginter, E., & Simko, V. (2016). New data on harmful effects of trans-fatty acids. *Bratislava Medical Journal, 117*(5), 251–253. https://doi.org/10.4149/bll_2016_048

Hu, Y., Hu, F. B., & Manson, J. E. (2019). Marine omega-3 supplementation and cardiovascular disease: An updated meta-analysis of 13 randomized controlled trials involving 127,477 participants. *Journal of the American Heart Association, 8*(19), e013543. https://doi.org/10.1161/JAHA.119.013543

Jennings, A., Cunnane, S. C., & Minihane, A. M. (2020). Can nutrition support healthy cognitive ageing and reduce dementia risk? *BMJ: British Medical Journal, 369*, m2269. https://doi.org/10.1136/bmj.m2269

Kheirouri, S., & Alizadeh, M. (2021). MIND diet and cognitive performance in older adults: A systematic review. *Critical Reviews in Food Science and Nutrition.* Advance online publication. https://doi.org/10.1080/10408398.2021.1925220

McGrattan, A. M., McGuinness, B., McKinley, M. C., Kee, F., Passmore, P., Woodside, J. V., & McEvoy, C. T. (2019). Diet and inflammation in cognitive ageing and Alzheimer's disease. *Current Nutrition Reports, 8*(2), 53–65. https://doi.org/10.1007/s13668-019-0271-4

Morris, M. C. (2016). Nutrition and risk of dementia: Overview and methodological issues. In *Annals of the New York Academy of Sciences: Vol. 1367. Nutrition in prevention and management of dementia* (pp. 31–37). New York Academy of Sciences. https://doi.org/10.1111/nyas.13047

Morris, M. C., Tangney, C. C., Wang, Y., Sacks, F. M., Barnes, L. L., Bennett, D. A., & Aggarwal, N. T. (2015). MIND diet slows cognitive decline with aging. *Alzheimer's and Dementia, 11*(9), 1015–1022. https://doi.org/10.1016/j.jalz.2015.04.011

Mozaffarian, D., Rosenberg, I., & Uauy, R. (2018). History of modern nutrition science-implications for current research, dietary guidelines, and food policy. *British Medical Journal, 361*, k2392. https://doi.org/10.1136/bmj.k2392

Porter, K., Hoey, L., Hughes, C. F., Ward, M., & McNulty, H. (2016). Causes, consequences and public health implications of low B-vitamin status in ageing. *Nutrients, 8*(11), 725. https://doi.org/10.3390/nu8110725

Tucker, J., Fischer, T., Upjohn, L., Mazzera, D., & Kumar, M. (2018). Unapproved pharmaceutical ingredients included in dietary supplements associated with US Food and Drug Administration warnings. *JAMA Network Open, 1*(6), e183337. https://doi.org/10.1001/jamanetworkopen.2018.3337

Zhang, E., Miller, D. D., & Li, W. (2021). Non-musculoskeletal benefits of vitamin D beyond the musculoskeletal system. *International Journal of Molecular Sciences, 22*(4), 2128. https://doi.org/10.3390/ijms22042128

# CHAPTER 6

# GET YOUR SHUT-EYE: SLEEP FOR A HEALTHY BRAIN

I watched with bated breath on July 30, 2020, when NASA's Mars Perseverance rover began its ascent into the atmosphere. As the unmanned spacecraft began its nearly 7-month journey to the red planet, I thought, "I can't believe I have a vested interest in this epic mission!" One of my many hats—and the one that surprises people the most— is NASA scientist. I was recruited to their behavioral health and performance research team to help get people safely to Mars!

If you're wondering what a neuropsychologist has to do with Mars exploration, you're in good company. The connection might not be intuitive, but it actually makes sense when you consider the challenges astronauts face during space travel. They spend long periods of time in near-isolation; in confined quarters; and in extreme environments that expose them to radiation, carbon dioxide, and microgravity. All of these conditions threaten health and well-being, including brain health. Cognitive problems—sometimes called "space fog"—and mood changes can jeopardize the mission and result in dire consequences. So, it is critical that we identify and try to minimize the risk of cognitive, physical, and mental health problems in astronauts. And this is where my expertise in brain health comes into play!

When I first began my position with NASA, I was surprised to learn that sleep disruption poses one of the greatest risks to the brain health of astronauts. In fact, sleep is one of the three research areas in NASA's Behavioral Health and Performance Element. The other two are behavioral medicine, which deals with mood, cognitive function, and other behavioral reactions to living and working in space; and team risk, which focuses on different aspects of team dynamics, such as crew cohesion and communication. During space flight, astronauts sleep less than they do on the ground, and the quality of their sleep is reduced. Because they lose the usual daytime–nighttime light cycle that we experience on earth, their circadian rhythms—the brain's internal clocks—are thrown off. And studies consistently show that, whether we're in space or on the ground, we need to get a good amount of quality sleep for our brains to function at peak levels.

This chapter breaks down the different types of sleep studies researchers conduct and summarizes what those studies have revealed about the powerful impact sleep has on the brain. You will learn how sleep changes with age and how it is linked to dementia. We will go over practical advice for how to sleep better and what to do if you have signs of a sleep disorder that requires medical attention.

## WHAT RESEARCH TELLS US

Scientists study the effects of sleep—or lack of sleep—on health using different techniques. One method is to give people questionnaires that ask about their sleep habits, such as how many hours of sleep they get on a typical night, how long it takes them to fall asleep, how often they wake up in the middle of the night, and how rested they feel during the day. This type of self-report measure is convenient, but it is limited by the fact that people have to be tuned in to their habits and feelings and must be honest when they respond to questionnaires. Other research methods can get around those issues but come with their own complications. In some studies, volunteers sleep in a research laboratory for one or more nights. This is great because the researchers can directly monitor their sleep but, as you might imagine, the very fact of sleeping in an unfamiliar place and knowing you are being watched can affect your sleep.

The most comprehensive type of sleep study in a research laboratory is called *polysomnography*. This type of study uses different medical devices to monitor changes in the body that typically happen during sleep. For example, an EEG, which stands for "electroencephalogram," measures brain waves, or electrical activity, in the brain. Sleep scientists might also measure the oxygen level in your blood, your heart rate and breathing, or eye and leg movements while you sleep. Great information about the amount and quality of sleep comes from these types of studies, but a big limitation is the fact that being hooked up to wires and monitors can disrupt sleep. Thanks to advances in technology, there are now a number of wearable sleep trackers, including wristbands, armbands, smart watches, and even rings, that collect much of the same data sleep researchers need, and in the comfort of your own home!

Regardless of the type of sleep study, research points in the same direction: Sleep is essential to health and well-being.

## The Quantity and Quality of Sleep Affect Health and Well-Being

We need sleep to support the functioning of all of our major body systems, including our immune, cardiovascular, metabolic, and endocrine systems. Sleep also supports different cognitive and emotional processes, such as our ability to focus our attention, to learn and remember information, to control our emotions, and to feel motivated. Studies have shown that sleeping an average of 7 to 8 hours each night is related to better brain health as well as better physical health. One of the keys to good sleep is to have a regular sleep–wake schedule, regular daily exposure to light, and regular physical activity. This helps keep our circadian rhythms on track. Getting enough good-quality sleep is vital to healthy living.

Unfortunately, sleep problems abound in the United States. About one third of Americans report insufficient regular sleep, which the Centers for Disease Control and Prevention defines as less than 7 hours per night. Results of an AARP survey paint an even bleaker picture of sleep patterns in later decades of life. They found that 43% of people in the United States age 50 years and older said they don't get enough sleep. Fifty-four percent wake up too early and can't get back to sleep, and 44% said they rarely or never sleep all night without waking up for more than a few minutes. We probably all know what it's like to toss and turn all night, or pull an all-nighter to cram for an exam, and then feel exhausted and cranky the next day. It can be hard to stay focused or motivated. These immediate effects of just one night of sleep deprivation are bad enough, but the consequences are even worse if we are chronically sleep deprived.

"Bad sleep generally results in bad wakefulness," Mohammad Nami told me over Zoom when we met to talk about his research on sleep and health. Nami is a Fellow at Harvard Medical School and an international expert in the field of sleep medicine. His statement succinctly captures what research tells us about the health effects of insufficient sleep. People who chronically get inadequate sleep are at risk for health problems ranging from heart disease, obesity, and diabetes to cancer and inflammatory disorders such as rheumatoid arthritis and irritable bowel syndrome. Sleep loss even makes us more sensitive to pain! Our immune system suffers when we are sleep deprived, making it harder for our body to fight off illnesses. Nami explained that lack of sleep can make us susceptible to viral infections because sleep loss disrupts the balance among different parts of our immune system. When we get insufficient sleep, three big changes happen in our immune system:

1. *Activity of our natural killer cells goes down.* Natural killer cells are a type of white blood cells that help the body fight off viral infections.
2. *Production of antibodies slows down.* These are proteins in the blood that recognize and neutralize foreign substances that enter the body, such as bacteria and viruses.
3. *Production of inflammatory cytokines goes up.* Cytokines are molecules that allow your cells to talk to each other and help your body fight off infections by directing the activity of the immune system. But too many cytokines can overwhelm your body, leading them to misdirect the immune system's activity.

These consequences of insufficient sleep on the immune system are an even greater concern in the time of the COVID-19 pandemic, when we are all at risk of being exposed to a dangerous virus. Complicating this picture, anxiety—which has been heightened in most of us during the pandemic—not only can weaken our immune system on its own but also interferes with sleep, which further weakens our immune system.

Chronic lack of sleep also affects our brains in different ways. Science tells us that *restricted sleep* (not getting enough sleep) or *disrupted sleep* (waking up often and therefore getting short periods of sleep) is linked to the following:

- A smaller hippocampus, the brain region we have discussed multiple times because of its critical role in memory.
- Thinning in the cerebral cortex, which is the folded, outer layer of the brain.

- An increase in the size of the ventricles, the spaces in the brain that are filled with cerebrospinal fluid. This is a bad thing because enlarged ventricles are a warning sign that the brain is getting smaller.
- Reduced *neurogenesis*, which is the process of forming new brain cells.
- Disrupted and inefficient communication between different parts of the brain.

As you might expect based on how sleep deprivation affects the brain, sleep problems are also associated with cognitive problems. Strong scientific evidence for this relationship comes from a meta-analysis that combined the findings from 51 different longitudinal studies of sleep and cognitive decline. When the researchers analyzed patterns across all 51 studies, they found that people with sleep problems were at greater risk of experiencing cognitive decline over time compared with people who generally sleep well. Different characteristics of sleep, such as having trouble falling asleep, staying asleep, or functioning during the day because of fatigue, were important. The studies included in the meta-analysis used self-report questionnaires to measure sleep, but studies that used other methods, such as polysomnography, or monitoring changes in the body during sleep with medical devices, have shown the same patterns.

Some types of cognitive skills seem to be more vulnerable to sleep problems than others. Attention, short-term memory, mental speed, and executive functions suffer the most when we are sleep deprived. One type of attention, *vigilance*, is especially vulnerable. Vigilance is our ability to continuously maintain focus on a task for an extended period of time. Staying vigilant is extremely important for staying safe during everyday activities, such as driving. Some people have careers that also put heavy demands on vigilance, such as air traffic controllers, pilots, and astronauts! Their jobs require them to maintain attention for long periods of time and to pick up on fairly rare, but critical, events or stimuli. Take, for example, Captain "Sully" Sullenberger's quick response when a bird unexpectedly struck the plane he was piloting and disabled the engines; he somehow was able to safely land US Airways Flight 1549 in the Hudson River. Unfortunately, many of these professionals are also more likely to be sleep deprived, which brings us back to the NASA example that started off this chapter. Studies show that sleep deprivation has immediate effects on vigilance, slowing reaction time and increasing lapses in attention during tasks that require vigilance. Vigilance goes down after a night of total sleep deprivation, but it can even go down after several nights of getting 5 hours or less of sleep per night. This can lead to fatal consequences. For example, drowsy driving causes thousands of automobile crashes every year, according to the National Highway Traffic Safety Administration (https://www.nhtsa.gov/risky-driving/drowsy-driving).

## Sleep Changes as You Age

There is some debate about whether we need less sleep as we grow older, but the general consensus is that the need for sleep does not change with age. However, the quality and quantity of our sleep change as we grow older. We tend to have more nighttime awakenings because we have less deep sleep, the stage of sleep when our body and brain slows down, which we need to feel refreshed when we wake up in the morning. We also become more vulnerable to disturbances during our sleep, such as sounds in our environment. Our body's internal clock shifts, and with that comes a change in the timing of sleep: As we age, we have more difficulty staying up late, so we tend to fall asleep earlier and, as a result, awake earlier in the morning. Deep sleep decreases from about our 30s to our 60s. Despite these changes, persistent, excessive sleepiness during the day is not a normal part of aging. In some people, persistent daytime sleepiness is a sign of a sleep disorder.

Sleep disorders, or medical conditions that affect your ability to get enough good-quality sleep, become more common with age. According to large studies that calculate the rates of different diseases, insomnia afflicts almost 50% of older adults—a rate more than double what we see in young adults. *Insomnia* is a medical disorder that is marked by problems falling asleep, staying asleep, or waking up too early and being unable to fall back to sleep, at least 3 nights per week for at least 3 months. Sleep-disordered breathing—an umbrella term that describes different conditions that affect how we breathe during sleep—also increases with age. Perhaps the best-known example is *sleep apnea*, a condition in which breathing repeatedly stops and starts during sleep, often causing loud snoring, which results in poor-quality sleep. Sleep disorders such as insomnia and sleep apnea can lead to more severe cognitive and brain changes than occasional sleep difficulties. Fortunately, sleep disorders are treatable, as we discuss later in this chapter.

## Sleep Problems Are Linked to Dementia

In 2019, researchers at the Martinos Center for Biomedical Imaging at Massachusetts General Hospital published the results of a fascinating study. Volunteers in the study allowed researchers to take pictures of their brains and record electrical activity from their brains while they slept. Yes, the researchers were able to find a group of people who managed to sleep inside a noisy brain scanner! The volunteers wore an EEG cap while they slept so the researchers could measure their brain waves. The results showed that brain waves that appear when a person enters deep sleep were followed seconds later by alternating waves of blood and cerebrospinal fluid in the brain. *Cerebrospinal fluid* is a clear liquid that surrounds the brain and spinal cord, providing a cushion for those organs, picking up nutrients from the blood, and clearing the brain of toxic waste. Some of the toxins that cerebrospinal fluid washes away are associated with Alzheimer's disease. It follows that sleep deprivation interferes with this waste clearance, which in turn can increase the risk for Alzheimer's disease. And this is exactly what other researchers have shown.

In one study, scientists gave older adults a special type of brain scan that showed the beta-amyloid protein, one of the brain markers of Alzheimer's disease. People in the study also completed a questionnaire about the quality of their sleep. The adults who had the most problems falling asleep at night were the ones who had the most beta-amyloid protein in their brain. Studies also have shown that older adults who wake up often in the middle of the night—what researchers describe as *fragmented sleep*—have a higher risk of Alzheimer's disease and other types of dementia than older adults who sleep soundly. Scientists have even found that sleep problems during mid-life can increase the risk for dementia decades later, which fits with the idea that we need sleep to protect the brain from building up the toxic waste that can cause different forms of dementia.

Not only can sleep problems increase your risk for dementia, but dementia also can interfere with sleep patterns. People with Alzheimer's disease tend to wake up more in the middle of the night, and they are often disoriented when they wake up. This can cause them to sleep more during the day. Dementia often disrupts circadian rhythms, which, combined with cognitive impairment, can lead to confusion about when it's daytime and when it's nighttime. Sleep problems in dementia increase the risk of complications, such as agitation and aggression, and speed up the rate of cognitive decline.

We need enough good-quality sleep to maintain the healthiest brain possible, whether or not we have dementia, whether we're young or in our older years, and whether we're in good physical health or dealing with health problems. So, let's talk about how to sleep well!

## SLEEP WELL! IMPROVING YOUR SLEEP HABITS FOR A HEALTHY BRAIN

To improve your sleep, keep healthy sleep habits that can help you fall asleep and stay asleep—what health professionals call good *sleep hygiene*. Sleep expert Dr. Nami summarized tips for sleep hygiene in five categories.

First is *timing*. Try to have a regular sleep–wake schedule. That means you should go to sleep at night and get up in the morning around the same time each day. Consistency is key to good sleep hygiene. Avoid taking naps. Experts from the Global Council on Brain Health suggest that if you must nap, you should limit the nap to 30 minutes in the early afternoon.

Second is *sleep behavior*. Follow a regular routine in preparation for bedtime every night to signal to your body and mind that bedtime is approaching. Your routine might include spending 15 minutes or so to prepare for the next day; taking care of basic hygiene, such as washing your face and brushing your teeth; and ending with an activity to wind down, such as reading, listening to relaxing music, or praying. Go to bed only when you feel drowsy enough to fall asleep. If you aren't able to fall asleep after about 15 minutes, find a place to relax outside of bed—perhaps go back to one of the relaxing activities that help you wind down. Return to bed only once you feel sleepy. Limit external stimulation, and limit activity in your bed besides sleep, such as watching TV, reading, or using your smartphone or tablet. Avoid difficult discussions or arguing while you're winding down for the night.

The third category of tips for good sleep hygiene is *environment*. Create a physical environment that promotes good, restful sleep. Keep the bedroom quiet and dark at night. Maintain a bedroom temperature that is comfortable to you, perhaps slightly cooler than usual. Take a warm bath and put on comfortable pajamas. If it helps, wear earplugs or an eye mask to shield yourself from external stimulation.

Number four is *ingestion*. Think about what you put in your body in the evening hours. Avoid heavy meals or stimulating drinks, such as coffee or tea, late in the evening. If you need an evening snack, opt for something light and healthy. Limit your alcohol late at night. Even though alcohol might help you fall asleep, research shows that it interferes with the quality of sleep—you are more likely to wake up during the night, and your usual cycle of sleep stages can be disrupted.

The fifth and final category is *mental control*. Avoid stimulating activities, such as vigorous exercising. Instead, choose mentally quiet activities such as low-impact stretching or relaxation strategies, which we discuss more in the next section. As Nami put it, "Enjoy the power of silence." Do what will help you find a sense of tranquility and harmony.

## Set Daytime Habits to Get the Optimal Amount of Sleep at Night

Set a goal of getting 7 to 8 hours of solid, uninterrupted sleep each night. The Global Council on Brain Health and other experts suggest that this is the sweet spot for maintaining good physical and cognitive health. Quite a few studies, including a recent meta-analysis, show that it's not only getting too little sleep that puts our brains at risk, but also too much sleep! Studies have shown a link between sleeping 9 or more hours per night and cognitive impairment in older adults. "Sleep is a Goldilocks issue: both too much and too little aren't good. Aim for 'just right,'" as a Harvard Health blog put it (LeWine, 2020).

Many people turn to medications or supplements to help them get more sleep. In general, try to avoid using over-the-counter medications for sleep because they can have negative side effects, in particular as we get older. Your health care provider might prescribe medication for sleep if you have a sleep disorder, but make sure to get clear instructions about how often you should use them. Studies show that habitual use can limit their effectiveness, so you might want to consider limiting their use to three nights during the week, unless your health provider says otherwise. Some people benefit from dietary supplements for sleep, such as melatonin, but keep in mind that the scientific evidence on their effectiveness is inconclusive.

There are things you can do during the day to help you sleep better at night. Exercising regularly—another key to good brain health—promotes good sleep. Expose yourself to light during the day. Light helps us establish a healthy sleep cycle, so maximizing exposure to bright light during the day and minimizing exposure to light at night can improve our sleep. Natural sunlight is best, so try to spend some time outdoors without sunglasses during the day. This is a great opportunity to combine sleep hygiene with exercise: Go for a walk, take a hike, or ride a bicycle during the day to get some exercise and expose yourself to natural light at the same time! Exercising outdoors is a win–win situation for brain health. Throughout the day, sit near windows when you can, to get a boost from the sunlight filtering in. When outdoor sunlight isn't an option, bright indoor light can still be beneficial. Phototherapy lamps and indoor light enhancements help to adjust our circadian rhythms and can even treat depression!

As with any lifestyle change, take it one step at a time as you work on improving your sleep. There are a lot of recommendations, so it might seem daunting to take them all on at once. See this as a gradual process of improving one or more sleep habits week by week. The worksheet in Exhibit 6.1 gives you an example of how you can track your sleep hygiene each day of the week. Set a goal of

**EXHIBIT 6.1.** Sleep Hygiene Worksheet

| | | Sun | Mon | Tue | Wed | Thu | Fri | Sat |
|---|---|---|---|---|---|---|---|---|
| TIMING | Set a constant bed time | ☐ | ☐ | ☐ | ☐ | ☐ | ☐ | ☐ |
| | Set a constant wake time | ☐ | ☐ | ☐ | ☐ | ☐ | ☐ | ☐ |
| | Do not take naps | ☐ | ☐ | ☐ | ☐ | ☐ | ☐ | ☐ |
| SLEEP BEHAVIOR | Have a presleep ritual | ☐ | ☐ | ☐ | ☐ | ☐ | ☐ | ☐ |
| | Use the bed only for sleep | ☐ | ☐ | ☐ | ☐ | ☐ | ☐ | ☐ |
| | If unable to sleep for more than 15 minutes, get out of bed | ☐ | ☐ | ☐ | ☐ | ☐ | ☐ | ☐ |
| ENVIRONMENT | Take a warm bath | ☐ | ☐ | ☐ | ☐ | ☐ | ☐ | ☐ |
| | Keep temperature of room constant | ☐ | ☐ | ☐ | ☐ | ☐ | ☐ | ☐ |
| | Keep bedroom dark | ☐ | ☐ | ☐ | ☐ | ☐ | ☐ | ☐ |
| INGESTION | Avoid caffeine, nicotine, and alcohol before bed | ☐ | ☐ | ☐ | ☐ | ☐ | ☐ | ☐ |
| | Eat a light snack before bed | ☐ | ☐ | ☐ | ☐ | ☐ | ☐ | ☐ |
| MENTAL CONTROL | Avoid stimulating activities; do mentally quiet tasks | ☐ | ☐ | ☐ | ☐ | ☐ | ☐ | ☐ |
| | Use relaxation techniques (breathing, imagery) | ☐ | ☐ | ☐ | ☐ | ☐ | ☐ | ☐ |
| Total number of habits used per night: | | ☐ | ☐ | ☐ | ☐ | ☐ | ☐ | ☐ |

practicing at least one good sleep habit from each of the five categories every night. See if you can increase your total number of habits over the course of a month or two.

## Know the Difference Between Sleep Problems and a Sleep Disorder

We all go through periods when we're not getting enough good sleep. And in the hustle and bustle of modern life, many of us have come to accept limited or fitful sleep as an expected part of life. It's important to remember that sleep is an absolutely essential part of health, and we do not have to accept persistent sleep problems as inevitable. Setting and sticking to healthy sleep practices should be a priority. For some people, though, sleep continues to be an issue even when they try to maintain good sleep hygiene. In some cases, trouble sleeping may be a sign of a sleep disorder.

There are a variety of sleep disorders, such as insomnia; sleep-related breathing disorders; and *bruxism*, which is grinding or clenching your teeth during sleep. How can you know when your problems sleeping are signs of a disorder rather than the occasional difficulties we all experience? Nami suggested it might be time to see a specialist if you are not getting enough sleep and you "feel something isn't right." He highlighted these specific warning signs of a possible sleep disorder:

- persistent difficulties falling or staying asleep, especially when it affects your daytime functioning or well-being;
- problems waking up and getting going in the morning;
- difficulty staying awake during the day (e.g., feeling drowsy or fatigued, or having low energy);
- sleep that is not refreshing;
- issues with behavioral or emotional control (e.g., problems controlling your temper);
- trouble focusing, remembering, or thinking clearly (this is sometimes called *cognitive fog* or *brain fog*);
- body aches and soreness; and
- low motivation.

Look out for abnormal behaviors during sleep too, such as kicking, calling out or shouting, frequent nightmares, snoring, or acting out your dreams. Other symptoms that might signal a sleep disorder are waking up feeling short of breath, having uncomfortable sensations in your legs at bedtime, grinding your teeth, or waking up with a headache or aching jaws or ears.

Keep in mind that having one or more of these symptoms does not automatically mean that you have a sleep disorder, but if you experience them on a regular basis, it's worth getting checked out. This is especially true if the symptoms start to interfere with your social or work functioning. A health care provider can help you figure out whether you have a sleep disorder; whether something else is causing your problems, such as a medical condition, psychological disorder, or medication; or whether you're experiencing occasional sleep issues due to stress, your schedule, or short-term life circumstances that we all experience. Doctors and psychologists who specialize in sleep can recommend behavioral therapies, medications, or both. You don't have to accept chronic sleep problems as an unavoidable part of your life!

| Fall and Stay Asleep Better | | |
|---|---|---|
| Don't stay in bed if you are not sleepy | Do not spend too much time in bed awake | A regular warm bath may be beneficial 2–3 hours before bedtime |
| Wearing socks to bed may be beneficial if you have cold feet | Avoid difficult discussions or arguing in the evening | If you worry a lot in bed, schedule ~15 minutes in the a.m. as your "worry time" |
| Try relaxation therapies with deep breathing and meditation | Find your most comfortable position and sleep environment | Avoid long naps (no longer than 30 minutes in the early afternoon) |

*Note.* From "The Brain–Sleep Connection: GCBH Recommendations on Sleep and Brain Health," January 2017 (https://www.aarp.org/content/dam/aarp/health/brain_health/2017/01/gcbh-sleep-and-brain-health-report-english-aarp.doi.10.26419%252Fpia.00014.001.pdf). Copyright 2017 by the Global Council on Brain Health. Adapted with permission.

## Tips for Success

Embrace quietness for the best sleep. You can do this by practicing relaxation strategies, such as mindfulness meditation, and by disconnecting from electronic devices.

### CONSIDER MINDFULNESS AND OTHER RELAXATION STRATEGIES

In 1976, Harvard cardiologist Herbert Benson wrote a book with Miriam Klipper called *The Relaxation Response*. In it, they describe our ability to use our minds to encourage a physical state of deep rest. The authors termed this phenomenon the *relaxation response*, the opposite of the stress response that we, and other animals, experience when we are in situations we see as dangerous or threatening. This is basically the fight-or-flight response you might have heard of: As a survival mechanism, our bodies reflexively orchestrate a sequence of responses that can help us either fight off threat or flee to safety. Our stress hormones change, our heartbeat and breathing speed up, our muscles tense, and we start to sweat. The fight-or-flight response benefits us in the short term, but difficulty sleeping and other problems can happen when we either activate this response to stressors that are not truly life threatening, such as family conflict or pressure at work, or when our bodies stay in that zone after a threat is over, such as when someone develops posttraumatic stress disorder after being in a bad car accident.

The relaxation response is a way of countering the stress response. It involves intentionally slowing down our body and our mind. Using just the power of our mind, we can encourage our body to release chemicals and brain signals that slow our breathing, relax our muscles, and reduce our blood pressure. I find it amazing that we can use our mind to direct the body to slow down! Human beings have known this for millennia. There is evidence of people using meditation practices—a classic way to evoke the relaxation response—as early as 1500 B.C.E., but popularity in the Western world has skyrocketed in recent years. With that has come a surge of research showing the health benefits of meditation, especially what is called "mindfulness meditation": the practice of focusing on your breathing and being consciously aware of your thoughts, feelings, and bodily sensations at the present moment, without letting your attention wander into thoughts about the past or worries about the future. It is one of a variety of relaxation strategies that can change our physical and emotional responses to stress by promoting a physical state of deep rest. Some of the other strategies include deep breathing, focusing on a soothing word, using imagery to visualize tranquil scenes, repetitive prayer, yoga, and tai chi. Research shows that these strategies can be effective treatments for many stress related disorders, such as depression, high blood pressure, and pain. They can also help you fall asleep and stay asleep.

To get the most benefit out of using relaxation strategies for sleep, spend 20 minutes or so practicing mindfulness or another relaxation technique during the day. This will make it easier to bring yourself back into a state of relaxation when you try to go to sleep. It's also a great reprieve from the stressors of the day! There are a number of books, websites, and apps that can guide you through different relaxation techniques. Some examples are provided in the Resources and Suggested Readings section at the end of this chapter.

DISCONNECT!

We live in a connected world in which many of us—and I include myself!—spend most of our waking hours interacting with some type of electronic communication device. Whether we're checking emails on a computer, playing games on a tablet, or scanning text messages or social media on our cell phone, it's easy to continue our habits into the evening hours. In fact, at least half of American adults use technology in bed at least once a week, according to Suni (2021). In the same poll, nearly one third of people who responded said they use technology in bed every day, and one in five said they check their devices before going back to sleep when they wake up in the middle of the night. But all of this screen time can be counter-productive when it comes to sleep.

Digital screens, fluorescent lights, and LED lights emit what's called *blue light*, a short but high-energy wavelength in the light spectrum that is visible to humans. Research shows that blue light interferes with sleep by suppressing our brains from producing the hormone melatonin. Melatonin is important for sleep because it helps with the timing of our circadian rhythm, telling the body when it's time to sleep and when it's time to wake up. Exposure to blue light before bed can also limit how much time you spend in different stages of sleep. It reduces slow-wave and rapid eye movement sleep, both of which are important for cognitive functioning.

Aside from the negative effects of blue light, digital devices can interfere with sleep by keeping us mentally wired. This can be especially true when it comes to the behavior dubbed "doomscrolling." Doomscrolling refers to consuming an endless torrent of negative news through social media or other places online. The problem with doomscrolling is that it can reinforce negative thoughts, and research shows it is linked to greater anxiety, sadness, fear, and stress. This behavior can have a negative impact any time of day, but when we do it in the later evening hours, another result may be trouble falling asleep. But not only negative news keeps our brains from settling down for the night. Remember that any mentally stimulating activity can keep our body, and mind, from relaxing.

Try to disconnect from electronic devices at least 30 minutes before going to bed. If you do check your phone or other devices late at night, consider using the "nighttime mode" option that now comes on many devices. This mode automatically reduces blue light emissions and decreases the brightness on the device's screen. You can also manually dim the display or install an app on your device that filters out the blue/green wavelength at night if your device doesn't come with nighttime mode. If you work a night shift or have to be up late at night for other reasons, consider wearing blue light–blocking glasses, which are available at big box stores, sporting goods stores, and prescription glasses retailers.

## SUMMARY

Remember these key points about sleeping well to maintain a healthy brain:

- When we don't get enough sleep, we are at risk for a variety of health problems, including heart disease, diabetes, irritable bowel syndrome, and even cancer.
- Our immune system suffers when we are sleep deprived, which makes us susceptible to illness. Anxiety, which can cause or be caused by restricted sleep, can further weaken our immune system.
- Sleep problems can cause different parts of the brain to shrink and interrupt the production of new brain cells and communication between parts of the brain.
- People with sleep problems tend to have difficulties with cognitive functions, including attention, short-term memory, mental speed, and executive functions. Vigilance, our ability to continuously maintain focus on a task for an extended period of time, is especially vulnerable.
- As we grow older, we tend to have more nighttime awakenings, and we tend to fall asleep and awaken earlier than we did when

we were younger. We might also get less deep sleep and be at greater risk for sleep disorders.

- Sleep is important for clearing out toxins in our brain, including toxins that are linked to Alzheimer's disease. Sleep problems in mid-life or late life increase the risk of Alzheimer's disease and other types of dementia and, in turn, people who have dementia tend to have problems sleeping.

- To improve your sleep, practice good sleep hygiene. This includes paying attention to the timing of your sleep; your sleep behavior, such as having a regular bedtime routine; your physical environment; what you eat and drink in the evening hours; and your level of mental stimulation at night.

- Aim to get 7 to 8 hours of uninterrupted sleep each night, on average. Improve your chances of getting good, restful sleep by exercising and exposing yourself to light during the day and by disconnecting from electronic devices and practicing relaxation strategies, such as mindfulness meditation, before bed.

- See a physician or psychologist who specializes in sleep disorders if you're not sleeping well and have some of the warning signs of a sleep disorder, such as trouble functioning during the day because of fatigue, problems controlling your emotions, or snoring loudly. And be sure to consult your doctor about whether and how often you should take sleep medication.

## RESOURCES AND SUGGESTED READINGS

Global Council on Brain Health, "The Brain–Sleep Connection": https://www.aarp.org/content/dam/aarp/health/brain_health/ 2017/01/gcbh-sleep-and-brain-health-report-english-aarp.doi. 10.26419%252Fpia.00014.001.pdf

Science-based recommendations from an international group of brain experts to help you improve your sleep to boost brain health.

**Centers for Disease Control and Prevention, "Basics About Sleep":**
https://www.cdc.gov/sleep/about_sleep/index.html
Information about sleep disorders, how sleep affects health, and sleep recommendations for different age groups, including a link to a downloadable sleep diary.

Ameli, R. (2014). *25 lessons in mindfulness: Now time for healthy living.* American Psychological Association.
Practical, step-by-step guide to help you learn and practice mindfulness meditation. Includes information about the philosophy behind mindfulness and 25 lessons to guide you through mindfulness meditation.

**7 Best Sleep Apps for iPhone & Android:** https://www.sleepassociation.org/sleep-treatments/sleep-apps/
List of sleep apps recommended by the American Sleep Association.

**Breathe2Relax:**
App available on Apple (https://apps.apple.com/us/app/breathe2relax/id425720246) and Android (https://play.google.com/store/apps/details?id=org.t2health.breathe2relax&hl=en) devices
App designed by the National Center for Telehealth & Technology to teach breathing techniques that manage stress and promote relaxation. Completely free!

**CBT-i Coach:** https://mobile.va.gov/app/cbt-i-coach
App available on Apple or Android devices that gives a structured guide to improving sleep, including developing positive sleep routines, improving your sleep environment, and practicing mindfulness meditation.

**Headspace:** https://www.headspace.com/
One of the most popular mindfulness meditation apps, available for Apple or Android devices. Includes content specific to your

goals, such as falling asleep, meditating, or relieving stress. After a 7-day free trial, you can buy a monthly or yearly subscription.

## SELECTED REFERENCES

Bah, T. M., Goodman, J., & Iliff, J. J. (2019). Sleep as a therapeutic target in the aging brain. *Neurotherapeutics, 16*(3), 554–568. https://doi.org/10.1007/s13311-019-00769-6

Benson, H. (with Klipper, M. Z.). (1975). *The relaxation response.* Avon.

Chen, T. L., Chang, S. C., Hsieh, H. F., Huang, C. Y., Chuang, J. H., & Wang, H. H. (2020). Effects of mindfulness-based stress reduction on sleep quality and mental health for insomnia patients: A meta-analysis. *Journal of Psychosomatic Research, 135,* 110144. https://doi.org/10.1016/j.jpsychores.2020.110144

Christensen, M. A., Bettencourt, L., Kaye, L., Moturu, S. T., Nguyen, K. T., Olgin, J. E., Pletcher, M. J., & Marcus, G. M. (2016). Direct measurements of smartphone screen-time: Relationships with demographics and sleep. *PLOS ONE, 11*(11), e0165331. https://doi.org/10.1371/journal.pone.0165331

Dzierzewski, J. M., Dautovich, N., & Ravyts, S. (2018). Sleep and cognition in older adults. *Sleep Medicine Clinics, 13*(1), 93–106. https://doi.org/10.1016/j.jsmc.2017.09.009

Ettore, E., Bakardjian, H., Solé, M., Levy Nogueira, M., Habert, M. O., Gabelle, A., Dubois, B., Philippe, R., & David, R. (2019). Relationships between objectives sleep parameters and brain amyloid load in subjects at risk for Alzheimer's disease: The INSIGHT–preAD Study. *Sleep, 42*(9), zsz137. https://doi.org/10.1093/sleep/zsz137

Fultz, N. E., Bonmassar, G., Setsompop, K., Stickgold, R. A., Rosen, B. R., Polimeni, J. R., & Lewis, L. D. (2019, November 1). Coupled electrophysiological, hemodynamic, and cerebrospinal fluid oscillations in human sleep. *Science, 366*(6465), 628–631. https://doi.org/10.1126/science.aax5440

Goldberg, S. B., Tucker, R. P., Greene, P. A., Davidson, R. J., Wampold, B. E., Kearney, D. J., & Simpson, T. L. (2018). Mindfulness-based interventions for psychiatric disorders: A systematic review and meta-analysis. *Clinical Psychology Review, 59,* 52–60. https://doi.org/10.1016/j.cpr.2017.10.011

Gupta, R., Das, S., Gujar, K., Mishra, K. K., Gaur, N., & Majid, A. (2017). Clinical practice guidelines for sleep disorders. *Indian Journal of Psychiatry, 59*(Suppl. 1), S116–S138. https://doi.org/10.4103/0019-5545.196978

Irwin, M. R. (2019). Sleep and inflammation: Partners in sickness and in health. *Nature Reviews Immunology, 19*(11), 702–715. https://doi.org/10.1038/s41577-019-0190-z

Janku, K., Smotek, M., Farkova, E., & Koprivova, J. (2020). Block the light and sleep well: Evening blue light filtration as a part of cognitive behavioral therapy for insomnia. *Chronobiology International, 37*(2), 248–259. https://doi.org/10.1080/07420528.2019.1692859

Ji, X., & Fu, Y. (2021). The role of sleep disturbances in cognitive function and depressive symptoms among community-dwelling elderly with sleep complaints. *International Journal of Geriatric Psychiatry, 36*(1), 96–105. https://doi.org/10.1002/gps.5401

Krause, A. J., Simon, E. B., Mander, B, A,, Greer, S. M., Saletin, J. M., Goldstein-Piekarski, A. N., & Walker, M. P. (2017). The sleep-deprived human brain. *Nature Reviews Neuroscience, 18*(7), 404–418. https://doi.org/10.1038/nrn.2017.55

LeWine, H. E. (2020, June 15). *Too little sleep, and too much, affect memory.* Harvard Health Blog. https://www.health.harvard.edu/blog/little-sleep-much-affect-memory-201405027136

Ma, Y., Liang, L., Zheng, F., Shi, L., Zhong, B., & Xie, W. (2020). Association between sleep duration and cognitive decline. *JAMA Network Open, 3*(9), e2013573. https://doi.org/10.1001/jamanetworkopen.2020.13573

Mander, B. A., Winer, J. R., & Walker, M. P. (2017). Sleep and human aging. *Neuron, 94*(1), 19–36. https://doi.org/10.1016/j.neuron.2017.02.004

Mantua, J., & Simonelli, G. (2019). Sleep duration and cognition: Is there an ideal amount? *Sleep, 42*(3), zsz010. https://doi.org/10.1093/sleep/zsz010

Musiek, E. S., & Holtzman, D. M. (2016, November 26). Mechanisms linking circadian clocks, sleep, and neurodegeneration. *Science, 354*(6315), 1004–1008. https://doi.org/10.1126/science.aah4968

Nasrini, J., Hermosillo, E., Dinges, D. F., Moore, T. M., Gur, R. C., & Basner, M. (2020). Cognitive performance during confinement and sleep restriction in NASA's Human Exploration Research Analog

(HERA). *Frontiers in Physiology, 11*, 394. https://doi.org/10.3389/fphys.2020.00394

Nekliudov, N. A., Blyuss, O., Cheung, K. Y., Petrou, L., Genuneit, J., Sushentsev, N., Levadnaya, A., Comberiati, P., Warner, J. O., Tudor-Williams, G., Teufel, M., Greenhawt, M., DunnGalvin, A., & Munblit, D. (2020). Excessive media consumption about COVID-19 is associated with increased state anxiety: Outcomes of a large online survey in Russia. *Journal of Medical Internet Research, 22*(9), e20955. https://doi.org/10.2196/20955

Olaithe, M., Bucks, R. S., Hillman, D. R., & Eastwood, P. R. (2018). Cognitive deficits in obstructive sleep apnea: Insights from a meta-review and comparison with deficits observed in COPD, insomnia, and sleep deprivation. *Sleep Medicine Reviews, 38*, 39–49. https://doi.org/10.1016/j.smrv.2017.03.005

Sprecher, K. E., Bendlin, B. B., Racine, A. M., Okonkwo, O. C., Christian, B. T., Koscik, R. L., & Benca, R. M. (2015). Amyloid burden is associated with self-reported sleep in nondemented late middle-aged adults. *Neurobiology of Aging, 36*(9), 2568–2576. https://doi.org/10.1016/j.neurobiolaging.2015.05.004

Suni, E. (2021, June 21). *Technology in the bedroom.* OneCare Media. https://www.sleepfoundation.org/bedroom-environment/technology-in-the-bedroom

# CHAPTER 7

# TO YOUR HEALTH! MENTAL AND PHYSICAL WELLNESS FOR A HEALTHY BRAIN

As 2020 unfolded, scientists around the world mobilized, performing study after study to uncover the mysteries behind the new virus we now know as COVID-19. These research studies made it clear that the respiratory disease, which primarily manifests as a cough and a fever, comes along with a host of symptoms that initially surprised most of the public. Among those unexpected symptoms: neurological signs, such as a headache, loss of consciousness, and weakness in the arms and legs; and psychological symptoms, such as anxiety, insomnia, and depression.

COVID can infect brain cells, causing the cells to shrink or even die. It causes *neuroinflammation*, the process in which the brain's innate immune response is triggered by an injury, infection, or other harmful stimuli. Inflammation is a protective response that can be helpful in the short term but that can degrade the brain over time. COVID also affects the body's blood vessels, putting people at risk for complications such as high blood pressure and stroke.

Infection of brain cells, neuroinflammation, and damage to blood vessels may very well explain the neurological and psychiatric symptoms that afflict many who suffer from COVID. But scientists' understanding of the disease is evolving rapidly, so the explanation for these symptoms might be very different by the time you read this. One way or another, COVID gives us a prime example of the interplay among physical health, mental health, and brain health. There is a strong link between the health of the brain and medical conditions such as heart disease or multiple sclerosis, as well as psychological or mental health conditions such as depression and anxiety. Science tells us that we can achieve a healthier brain by treating medical and psychological disorders.

We are going to tackle a lot in this chapter. You will learn what science tells us about the links among physical health, mental health, and brain health. We will discuss how our physical environment affects all of these aspects of health and can make it harder for people in disadvantaged environments to maintain a healthy lifestyle. We will address the stigma of mental disorders that hinders many people from seeking mental health treatment, as well as financial and other barriers that limit medical treatment. And we'll go over tips, including ideas for how to overcome these barriers, so you can get the most out of your health care.

## WHAT RESEARCH TELLS US

Most of the clients who come to see me for a neuropsychological evaluation have a lot going on medically, and in many situations my conclusion is that their memory and cognitive difficulties stem from their medical conditions. Take, for example, a 63-year-old man who came to my clinic. Like most of my clients, this gentleman complained about his memory. He would read a news story and forget the information within 2 hours. He would make social plans or medical appointments and then quickly forget about them. His wife said that he asked her the same questions repeatedly, clearly forgetting that he had already asked, and that he was increasingly distracted during conversations.

It wasn't just his memory that was changing. Ever since he unexpectedly lost a very close friend in a tragic accident, about

2 years before I evaluated him, his mood had been completely different. He felt down, he wasn't interested in seeing friends or family, and he spent more and more time sleeping. He had fits of anger, which prompted him to take off in his truck to escape whatever situation was angering him. He also described feeling constantly "on edge" as well as anxious and worried most of the time. During my interview, I learned that he had used alcohol heavily for a long time but had stopped drinking for the past 15 years.

My client had an extensive history of heart disease. He had coronary artery disease, a condition in which cholesterol and fatty plaques build up in the arteries that supply blood to the heart, causing them to narrow or become blocked. He had suffered a heart attack in the past and had high blood pressure and high cholesterol.

Neuropsychological testing corroborated his memory complaints. He had difficulty when I asked him to learn a list of words or repeat short stories that I read to him. His mental speed was slower than expected, and his scores were low on tests that required him to use reasoning skills for solving problems or multitasking. I did not diagnose him with dementia—his cognitive difficulties were not severe enough, and they did not interfere with his daily activities. My conclusion was that his cognitive problems were caused by a combination of his heart disease, history of alcohol abuse, depression, and anxiety. Research tells us that each of these conditions can affect the brain and lead to problems with memory and cognitive skills. And for psychological conditions such as depression and anxiety, the reverse can also be true: Brain damage can actually be the cause of mental health problems.

## Heart Disease and Other Medical Conditions Can Affect Your Brain

When it comes to medical conditions that affect the brain, the biggest culprit is a group of illnesses that affect the blood supply in our bodies, called *heart disease* or *vascular disease*. As we learned earlier, vascular diseases can be *cardiovascular*, meaning they affect blood supply to the heart, or *cerebrovascular*, meaning they affect blood supply to the brain. Many vascular diseases are related to a condition called *atherosclerosis* that develops when a substance called *plaque* builds up in the walls of the arteries. Atherosclerosis can lead to coronary artery disease, as it did in my client we just learned about, and put you at risk for stroke, aneurysm, and other vascular diseases. Other examples of vascular diseases include congestive heart failure; peripheral artery disease; and transient ischemic attacks, sometimes called "mini-strokes." Behavior such as smoking and medical conditions such as high blood pressure, high cholesterol, diabetes, and obesity make it more likely that you will develop a vascular condition, so they are called *vascular risk factors*. Vascular diseases and vascular risk factors can affect the health of your brain, leading to cognitive and emotional problems.

Melissa Lamar is an expert on how vascular risk factors affect the brain and cognitive functioning as we age, so I talked to her, seeking insight into the link between vascular disease and brain health. Now at Rush University Medical Center, Lamar completed her postdoctoral fellowship right before me in the same lab at the National Institute on Aging, so in a way you can see her as my professional big sister. Her research builds on the decades of findings that tell us vascular risk factors in mid-life have a direct link to cognitive functioning in late life: People with uncontrolled blood pressure, high glucose, and other vascular risk factors in middle age tend to have faster rates of decline in their cognitive skills as they grow older. Lamar investigates what happens if you're already older—say, 65 or older—and have these same types of vascular risks. Through her research, she has found that older adults with vascular risk factors tend to have lower cognitive skills, similar to the pattern in mid-life. But the link is not as strong as what we see in middle-aged adults, which suggests that vascular conditions take their greatest toll before our senior years. This highlights how important it is to think about our overall health, and our brain health, *before* we hit our senior years, because what we do earlier in life sets the stage for how we age.

Vascular disease affects cognitive functioning because it interferes with blood flow throughout our body, and that includes the brain. Insufficient blood flow in the brain leads to different types of problems, including damage to the brain's *white matter*, the tissue in the brain containing bundles of nerve fibers that connect different regions in the brain together. White matter is essential for communication between parts of the brain. When that communication is disrupted, problems with different cognitive abilities occur, especially mental speed and executive functions. In some people, vascular disease causes so much damage to the brain that they develop a type of dementia called *vascular dementia*. People with vascular damage in their brains are also at risk for physical problems, such as impaired balance and falls, and for psychological disorders such as depression.

Aside from vascular disease, a variety of other physical conditions affect brain health. Research tells us that people with lung disease, HIV, kidney disease, and other medical disorders are at greater risk of cognitive impairment, mental disorders, and brain changes. Sensory changes, such as hearing loss, can also affect brain health. Several studies have shown that people with hearing loss, even at mild levels, perform worse on cognitive tests. Hearing loss has also been linked to a faster rate of brain atrophy in older adults and a greater risk of dementia. At the same time, sometimes changes in hearing or vision can be mistaken for cognitive impairment. If we can't hear well or see well, it becomes more difficult to remember what we have perceived. Someone with undiagnosed vision or hearing problems, or someone who is trying to mask their problems, might appear to have problems comprehending conversation or might seem disoriented or clumsy. These symptoms can raise fears of dementia or another brain disorder, but in many cases the issues are resolved once the hearing or vision problems are addressed. I have seen this often in my clinical practice. This highlights how important it is to stay on top of your physical health.

## Mental Disorders Can Be a Cause or Consequence of Brain Changes

My first experiences in the research world came in the late 1990s. I worked as a research assistant at the University of Texas Health Science Center at San Antonio during my senior year in college and the year after that. It was there that I learned about the link between depression and the brain, which set the stage for all of my research since. This was the time when neuroimaging research was really taking off as technological advances made it possible for scientists to use different types of scanners to peer into the brain and measure its structure and function. Doing so in people with psychological conditions such as depression allows us to see how the brain differs in people with and without those conditions and how different mental health treatments affect our brains.

Thanks to decades of this type of research, we now know that the brain is at the center of mental disorders, from depression to autism, from bipolar disorder to schizophrenia. Studies have shown that people with these conditions have brains that differ in size and function compared with people who do not have these conditions. For example, you learned in Chapter 4 that depressed people tend to have a smaller prefrontal cortex than their peers without depression and that depression interferes with the functioning of the prefrontal cortex and with the communication between the prefrontal cortex and other brain regions. Vascular disease is another way in which depression and the brain are linked. When vascular disease affects the brain's white matter, it interferes with networks of brain regions that are important for maintaining our mood, which can lead to depression. This is especially true in older adults because the risk for vascular disease rises the older we get.

Depression researchers face a chicken-and-the-egg problem: Which came first, depression or brain changes? The short answer is, both! Longitudinal studies that follow people over time show that you can predict changes in different brain regions on the basis of people's level of depressive symptoms at the beginning of the study, which suggests that depression came first. On the other hand, people who experience brain damage—for example, through a traumatic brain injury or a stroke—are more likely to become depressed in the future. So, it seems that brain changes came first in those instances. We call this a *bidirectional relationship* between depression and brain changes because each can cause the other.

My example focused on depression, but research tells us that a variety of psychological conditions are related to brain health. This is the reason I concluded that, in addition to vascular disease, the cognitive problems of the client we discussed earlier were caused by depression, anxiety, and substance abuse. The good news is that getting treatment for mental health problems can help you achieve a healthier brain! We'll come back to this later in the chapter.

## Our Physical Environment Affects Physical, Mental, and Brain Health

Physical health, mental health, and brain health affect each other. They are interrelated, so when one is affected, the others are often affected too. One way this plays out is in the effect of our physical environment on health. By "physical environment" I mean the neighborhoods where we live, work, learn, and play, and the resources those neighborhoods have to fulfill our basic needs. Neighborhoods determine the affordability and condition of the house we live in; the cleanliness of the air we breathe and the water we drink; the types of transportation we have access to; the quality of schools available to our families; the availability of green spaces, such as parks and trails; and the availability of nutritious food. Research shows that a clean, healthy environment is vital to physical health and emotional well-being. Lamar put it this way: "It's not just *how* you live, but it can also be *where* you live."

Where we live can either promote or limit our access to resources that support a healthy lifestyle that in turn helps us maintain a healthy brain. Much of Lamar's research focuses on understanding how factors such as physical environment, race, and income contribute to risk of vascular disease, dementia, and other illnesses that are more common as we grow older and that affect the health of our brains.

Socially disadvantaged groups often live and work in physical environments where it is harder to maintain a healthy lifestyle. This puts people at risk for medical conditions such as vascular disease and psychological conditions such as anxiety and depression, all of which can affect the brain. Lamar gave the example of how our physical environment affects nutrition. If you live in an area where there are no grocery stores nearby, and you don't have a car to drive to a grocery store in another area, then you are at the mercy of what is around you. In lower income areas, what is around you will mostly like be fast food restaurants or convenience stores, which typically don't sell fresh produce. This makes it harder to follow the Mediterranean-style diet we discussed in Chapter 5, for example. Another factor is the *walkability* of a neighborhood. In other words, how safe do you feel walking outside? Are there sidewalks in your neighborhood? Are there parks nearby? Research shows that the walkability of a neighborhood affects obesity and other aspects of health. All these aspects of physical environment can increase the risk of vascular diseases, depression, dementia, and other illnesses.

It's important to recognize how our environment affects health. On a societal level, we can continue to push for programs and services that reduce barriers that are preventing some of us from achieving optimal health. On an individual level, Lamar suggested, "We should talk to our doctor not just about how we feel but also where we live." If your physician or another health care provider recommends that you take a course of action to address a health issue, such as improving your diet or exercising more, be open about how feasible it is to follow through with the recommendations, given where you live. Explain why it might be hard for you to do what they're recommending. They can help you find opportunities and resources to overcome those barriers or refer you to a social worker or other professional who can help you find creative ways to stay as healthy as possible regardless of your physical environment.

## BE WELL! IMPROVING YOUR PHYSICAL AND MENTAL HEALTH FOR A HEALTHY BRAIN

My client who I described earlier is a great example of the interplay among physical health, mental health, and brain health. He didn't have dementia, but he did have problems with his memory, mental speed, and reasoning skills that seemed to be caused by a combination of medical and psychological conditions. My recommendations for him centered on getting treatment for these conditions. What's great is that many of the behaviors I recommend to my clients for physical and mental health are the very same behaviors you have already learned about for achieving and maintaining a healthy brain!

Let's break this down to better illustrate my point. After my assessment, my primary goals for this client were to improve his cognitive functioning, his mental health, and his vascular health. Because his physical and psychological problems were deemed the cause of his cognitive impairment, I expected that by treating those conditions, the impairment would improve too. For his vascular health, I suggested that he adopt a heart-healthy diet, increase his physical activity, and follow up with his cardiologist about medical treatment for his heart disease. All of these recommendations for his vascular health are also healthy behaviors we've learned about in this book to maintain a healthy brain. The same is true for most of my recommendations for his mental health. In addition to starting therapy, I suggested that he exercise, reconnect with his social network, and find some type of meaningful activity, such as volunteering, to keep his mind active. These are all great for our brains as well!

Getting help for medical conditions, whether physical or mental in nature, is essential to maintaining a healthy brain. You are already taking a step in the right direction by reading this book and learning how to reduce your risk for health problems, which improves what experts call *health literacy*. Health literacy is our ability to find, understand, and use health information to help us make medical decisions for our own health or the health of someone we love. In her research, Lamar has found that increasing health literacy is one way to improve vascular health in older adults who are trying to manage their vascular risk factors, such as high blood pressure, diabetes, and high cholesterol. Her research shows that the more someone knows about the link between heart health and healthy behaviors, such as a Mediterranean-style diet and exercise, the better they manage their vascular risk factors. Health literacy improves the outlook for physical health problems, but for most people, *mental* health literacy tends to lag behind physical health literacy. To achieve the healthiest brain possible, we must recognize, manage, and prevent both physical and psychological conditions.

**Let Go of Stigma and See a Mental Health Professional**

There are a lot of reasons why people don't seek medical or mental health treatment when they need it. Aside from lack of awareness about symptoms and treatment options, the high cost of care, lack of insurance or inadequate insurance, and lack of access to services can create barriers. Another big barrier is stigma, especially when it comes to treatment for mental health problems. *Stigma* refers to negative attitudes and beliefs, and in the case of mental health, stigma leads to fear and rejection of people with mental disorders. Because of that stigma, some people are reluctant to seek treatment for mental health concerns, as Angela Bethea-Walsh shared with me. Bethea-Walsh is a counseling psychologist in Atlanta, Georgia, who owns a clinical practice and provides therapy services for clients in my brain health company, CerebroFit. She pointed out that sometimes stigma is tied to culture. Cultural beliefs can create a feeling that seeking treatment means airing dirty laundry, shaming the family, or even betraying the family. Some cultures see mental health prob lems as a sign of personal weakness rather than disorders that have a strong basis in our genes and in the health and functioning of our body, similar to medical conditions.

Fortunately, attitudes about mental health are changing in the United States, according to a recent survey conducted by the Harris Poll on behalf of the American Psychological Association. According to the poll, 87% of American adults agree that having a mental health disorder is nothing to be ashamed of. Unfortunately, the same poll showed that 33% of Americans do not consider anxiety to be a mental disorder, and 22% do not consider depression to be a mental disorder (see https://www.apa.org/news/press/releases/apa-mental-health-report.pdf). In reality, depression and anxiety are the most common psychological disorders, and, as we have learned, they affect brain health. The important thing is that they are *treatable*, but treatment happens only if we acknowledge that they are a problem.

How do you know when your experiences signal a problem? We all have times when we feel sad or anxious, lack motivation, or stop enjoying the things we usually enjoy. This can be part of the ups and downs of normal life, but when the symptoms become severe, or start to interfere with your functioning at work, at home, or in your relationships, then it might be time to see a professional. Research shows that most people with mental health concerns seek treatment from their primary care doctor, but there are specialists with expertise in the diagnosis and treatment of psychological disorders. Some of the more common specialists include:

- *Psychologists*, who typically have a Doctor of Philosophy (PhD) or Doctor of Psychology (PsyD) degree, plus a state license to provide psychological services. There are different types of psychologists depending on the exact focus of their graduate school training, including clinical psychologists, counseling psychologists, and school psychologists. All of these types of psychologists provide psychotherapy, also called "talk therapy," to treat psychological disorders.

- *Psychiatrists*, who have a Doctor of Medicine (MD) or Doctor of Osteopathic Medicine (DO) degree and a medical license. Some psychiatrists provide psychotherapy, but their approach generally focuses on biomedical treatments, which are medications and medical procedures designed to reduce symptoms of psychological disorders. Medical procedures are typically reserved for people with severe symptoms that don't improve with medication or psychotherapy. This can include procedures called *brain stimulation therapies*, which use small amounts of electricity to either activate or inhibit parts of the brain that are dysfunctional. The type that most people have heard of is *electroconvulsive therapy*, or *ECT*, but there are others, including transcranial magnetic stimulation and transcranial direct current stimulation. The Resources and Suggested Readings section at the end of this chapter gives you links to websites that explain these types of treatments in greater detail.

- *Mental health counselors, licensed social workers, licensed professional counselors, and licensed marriage and family therapists*, who typically have a Master of Science (MS) or Master of Arts (MA) degree plus a license to provide mental health services. Similar to psychologists, their treatments usually focus on psychotherapy.
- *Advanced psychiatric nurses*, who hold a master's degree or higher in psychiatric–mental health nursing. They can provide psychotherapy, medication, or both, depending on the regulations in the state where they practice.

Your primary care doctor or other provider might refer you to one or more of these professionals. If you have concerns about your mental health; don't hesitate to ask! You are your own best advocate when it comes to your health care.

## Remember That One Size Does Not Fit All

Choosing to start therapy and finding a therapist can be intimidating and may take some time, which can cause frustration. Bethea-Walsh pointed out that "not every therapist is for everybody" and compared finding a therapist to buying jeans: You might try on a pair of jeans at the store and think they feel good and look good, but then you get home and they don't feel quite right any more, so you have to go back and try again. But you wouldn't give up on buying new jeans because the first pair didn't work out. The same can be said for finding a therapist. Each therapist is different, and not everyone will be a good fit for you. But don't stop looking.

You can look for therapists in your area using the variety of online resources that are available, some of which are listed at the end of this chapter. For example, the American Psychological

Association hosts a Psychologist Locator website (https://locator. apa.org/) where you can search for psychologists on the basis of your zip code, and most insurance providers allow you to search for mental health providers covered by your plan.

Bethea-Walsh also suggested that as you look for a therapist, think about who you would want to work with. Are you looking for a particular location (e.g., close to work vs. close to home)? Do you have a preference for the sex, race, or age group of a potential therapist? Do they accept your insurance, or do you need to pay out of pocket? You might also consider the person's specialty. For example, Bethea-Walsh specializes in therapy for people with a history of trauma or substance abuse, so someone with those concerns might seek her out in particular. Once you've found some options that seem appealing, remember that you can ask questions to help you decide if they're a good fit.

Some therapists, such as Bethea-Walsh, provide a free consultation visit, which gives you the chance to learn more about them and see whether they seem to be a good fit. She mentioned that some of the common questions she gets during the consultation visit are about finances, insurance coverage, availability for appointments at different times, and clinical approach. *Clinical approach*, also called *theoretical orientation*, refers to the therapist's philosophy about how problems develop and the techniques they use to treat those problems. For example, someone who uses a cognitive behavioral approach to therapy believes that negative thoughts are at the root of mental health problems, so they will help you recognize and challenge inaccurate, negative thoughts that feed depression, anxiety, and other psychological symptoms. Someone who conducts person-centered therapy will instead focus on your ability to reach your potential. Their techniques will center on being genuine and empathic so that they can build a relationship with you that will help you to grow. These approaches are very different, but research shows that both can be effective. There are lots of other approaches, and many therapists use techniques from more than one. But you might find some of these approaches to be off-putting, or you might simply find that you don't click with a therapist on a personal level. Don't give up! There are many options available, so keep looking until you find a good fit.

**Get the Most Out of Your Medical Treatment**

When it comes to treating medical conditions, my biggest piece of advice is to be an active consumer of your health care. That means a few different things, such as the following:

- If you have access to health care, use it! Don't hesitate to see your doctor if you notice new physical or psychological symptoms or if old symptoms get worse. In many situations, hesitating to talk to a health care provider makes the situation worse because the underlying condition progresses as more time passes without treatment.
- Again, ask questions! If anything your health care provider tells you isn't clear, don't be afraid to ask them to explain. You can also ask for take-home information, such as handouts, pamphlets, or brochures about your condition, or ask if they can recommend a reputable website that you can look up later to get more information. And don't hesitate to take notes during your visit. It can be difficult to remember details later, but the details are often important, so set yourself up for success by writing things down.
- Get a second opinion or ask for a referral to a specialist if you need to. Most of us see our primary care doctor as the first stop for our health care, but sometimes a specialist is more appropriate. For example, if your blood pressure or heart rate is out of control, you should probably see a cardiologist, or if you're having problems with balance or tingling in your

limbs, you might need to see a neurologist. Your primary care doctor can help determine what type of specialist you should see, but, as always, take the initiative to ask about seeing a specialist if you think you need one.

You will also get more out of your health care if you make sure your care is coordinated. This means that you have at least one doctor who knows everything that is happening with you medically. If you see another doctor, a psychologist, or any other health care provider, the coordinating doctor, who is usually your primary care doctor, should know about it and, when possible, have access to the medical records from your other providers. This allows your health care to be safer. For example, you can avoid overmedication when your doctor knows everything you are taking, even if some of your medications were prescribed by other providers. Coordinated care can also make your health care more effective because your doctor will have a more complete picture of your health.

## Tips for Success

It takes time to make changes for our physical and mental health, so be patient with yourself as you take things step by step and think creatively about ways to overcome barriers. Try to adopt healthy behaviors before health problems arise or worsen.

### TAKE IT ONE STEP AT A TIME

Working on our physical and mental health takes time and effort, like all of the healthy behaviors we have discussed in this book. And it might feel overwhelming if you get a long list of recommendations from your doctor or therapist about the changes you should make to improve your health. Be patient with yourself. Change will not happen overnight. Lamar, the neuropsychologist and vascular disease expert, offered some great advice about improving your health. Let's say that your doctor gives you 10 suggestions for controlling your blood pressure, such as losing weight, exercising regularly, reducing salt in your diet, and so on. Lamar's advice is "Slowly chip away at it . . . because trying to change 10 things all at the same time is pretty hard." And sometimes, if we take on too much, nothing gets done at all. She suggests that instead, you pick one thing you can really focus on: "Do it, make it a habit, then come back to the list and find that next thing that you want to work on." She also suggests that you talk to your doctor about the best course of action. If they give you lots of different changes to make, ask them what they're most worried about or what they see as the most important behavior to change, and that can be the one thing you start with. This doesn't mean that you won't get to the other recommendations, just that you will make change more manageable by taking it one step at a time.

Along the same lines, take things one step at a time when it comes to your mental health. Getting better takes time. If you are prescribed medication, it's common to try a few different medications before finding one that works for you. If you choose to go to therapy, it takes time to build a relationship with your therapist, get to the root of your issues, and begin the process of change. Therapy can unearth pain that is difficult to discuss. Sometimes people in therapy feel worse before they feel better as they open up old wounds to begin the process of properly healing. Even with these challenges, the investment of your time, energy, and emotions are worth it in the end when you improve your mental health.

TRY TO OVERCOME BARRIERS

We have already discussed stigma, but there are other barriers that can get in the way when we try to improve our physical and mental health. A major barrier can be cost. Affordability limits access to health care for many, especially those who are uninsured or underinsured, meaning they have insurance but their benefits do not cover the full expense of their claims. Unfortunately, these issues disproportionately affect some groups more than others, such as Black and Brown people and people in rural communities. Medicare can help if you are 65 years or over. Benefits cover both physical and mental health care. If you are eligible for Medicaid, you can also receive benefits for physical and mental health services. There are a variety of organizations that offer financial assistance, low-cost prescriptions, sliding fee scales based on income, and other services to improve access to affordable health care. You can find information about some of these resources at the end of this chapter.

Distrust of health care providers and the medical system as a whole creates barriers, too, and unfortunately this is another issue that has the greatest impact on groups that are already vulnerable, such Black and Brown people, LGBTQ people, and people from low-income households. A lot of changes must be made in the health care system to foster trust in the groups that are affected by biases and discrimination in the system and by individual providers. If distrust is a barrier for you, I encourage you to look for a provider you feel comfortable with, and keep looking if you're not happy with your current provider. Some people find it helpful to have a doctor or therapist from their own cultural group. You can search online for information about a potential doctor's or therapist's record of working with members of your group.

It can be helpful to think about barriers and how you might overcome them. Some of the more common barriers and possible solutions are described in the "Barriers to Treatment and Possible Solutions" graphic in the next section.

PRACTICE PREVENTION

Have you ever heard "An ounce of prevention is worth a pound of cure" or "Prevention is the best medicine"? These sayings apply to our physical health, our mental health, and our brain health.

## BARRIERS TO TREATMENT AND POSSIBLE SOLUTIONS

### LIMITED FINANCES OR LACK OF INSURANCE COVERAGE

Check to see if you qualify for government health care assistance, such as Medicaid, Medicare, or veterans' benefits, which can help with both medical and psychological treatment. If you have insurance, call your insurance company to see what services are covered. For psychotherapy, shop around for lower fees, and ask if the potential therapist provides services on a sliding fee scale (based on income) or if they offer any reduced-fee or pro bono services. Check nonprofit agencies and county programs, which often offer services to help with financial barriers. Dial 211 to reach a referral specialist who can connect you with medical and mental health services, including free support groups and other low-cost options.

### LACK OF TRANSPORTATION

Consider public transportation if it is available in your area. Many communities offer transportation services for people who don't have transportation or are unable to drive, such as volunteer driver programs, transportation voucher programs, and escort services. Go to https://eldercare.acl.gov/ to find transportation services in your local community. Ask if the hospital or clinic provides shuttle services. Ask your provider about telehealth options that will allow you to have therapy sessions or doctor's appointments by computer or over the phone.

### DISTRUST OF HEALTH CARE PROVIDERS

Try to find health care providers you are comfortable with. It's OK to find another doctor or therapist if you aren't happy with the one you have. In therapy, research shows that the relationship between the therapist and client is crucial to making progress, so make it a priority to work with someone you feel you can trust. Ethnic and racial minorities, sexual and gender minorities, and people from other marginalized groups often feel greater distrust of health care providers based on past discrimination and mistreatment. It might help to find a provider from the same group or do your research to learn about your potential provider's attitude toward or experience working with marginalized groups (many therapists make statements about this on their website).

### GEOGRAPHICAL LIMITATIONS

Consider telehealth, which is not location dependent. Many medical and mental health care providers have opened up their practices to telehealth out of necessity during the COVID-19 pandemic, and undoubtedly this will continue to be offered once the pandemic ends. Telehealth can include video or phone consultations and is available in both urban and rural areas. Talk to your provider if you have limited access to high-speed internet or a private place to talk, which can be an obstacle for telehealth appointments.

As much as we need to seek treatment when we have problems, it's even better if we can prevent the problems to begin with. Fortunately, as we have already learned, many of the healthy behaviors that treat or prevent problems in one area of health benefit other aspects of health as well. For example, if you get regular exercise and maintain a healthy diet earlier in life, you can lower your risk of heart disease, depression, and dementia in your golden years. Health is a lifelong process. Don't wait until you already have health problems to start living a healthy lifestyle. If possible, adopt healthy habits before you notice problems with your physical, emotional, or cognitive functioning. Taking steps to prevent health problems does not guarantee that we won't go on to develop medical or psychological conditions, but at the very least it can give us our best shot at staying healthy and happy longer.

## SUMMARY

Remember these key points about managing your physical and mental health to maintain a healthy brain:

- Physical health, mental health, and brain health are interrelated. Medical conditions and psychological conditions can affect your brain, and brain changes can also lead to different physical and psychological conditions. To achieve the healthiest brain possible, we must recognize, manage, and prevent both physical and psychological conditions.
- Vascular conditions and vascular risk factors affect blood supply to the body, including the brain. These conditions are linked to worse cognitive functioning, dementia, and depression. Mid-life is an especially important time for treating these conditions to prevent problems in later life.
- The brain is at the center of mental disorders. For example, changes in the brain can increase your risk of depression, and the reverse is also true: Depression can cause brain changes.

- Our physical environment, where we live, work, learn, and play, can either promote or limit our access to resources that support the sort of healthy lifestyle that helps us maintain a healthy brain. Talk to your doctor if your physical environment makes it hard for you to follow medical recommendations.

- When sadness, anxiety, or other psychological symptoms become severe, or start to interfere with your functioning, consider seeing a psychologist or other mental health specialist. Look for a therapist you feel comfortable with, and don't give up if things don't work out with the first therapist you try.

- Be proactive about seeing a health care provider if you have physical or mental health concerns. Don't be afraid to ask questions, and make sure to take notes. Get a second opinion or ask for a referral to a specialist if you need to.

- Working on our physical and mental health takes time and effort. Take things one step at a time.

- Identify barriers to seeking treatment, such as stigma, limited finances, or transportation, and think of ways to overcome them. Ask your health care provider for guidance if you need to.

- Remember that prevention is the best medicine. All the lifestyle behaviors you've learned not only help you maintain a healthy brain but also help prevent or treat many medical and psychological conditions.

## RESOURCES AND SUGGESTED READINGS

Global Council on Brain Health, "The Brain–Heart Connection": https://www.aarp.org/content/dam/aarp/health/brain_health/2020/02/gcbh-heart-health-report-english.doi.10.26419-2Fpia.00099.001.pdf

A brief summary of scientific evidence and useful advice for keeping a healthy heart for a healthy brain.

**Global Council on Brain Health, "Brain Health and Mental Well-Being":** https://www.aarp.org/content/dam/aarp/health/brain_health/2018/11/gcbh-mental-well-being-report-english.doi.10.26419-2Fpia.00037.001.pdf

Information from a group of international brain experts on boosting your mental well-being as a way of maintaining a healthy brain.

**National Institute on Aging, "Talking With Your Doctor":** https://www.nia.nih.gov/health/doctor-patient-communication/talking-with-your-doctor

Collection of articles to help you make the most of your doctor's appointments by being prepared, asking questions, and tracking your medications.

**National Institute on Aging, "Brain Stimulation Therapies":** https://www.nimh.nih.gov/health/topics/brain-stimulation-therapies/brain-stimulation-therapies.shtml

Overview of treatments for psychological conditions that involve activating or inhibiting activity in the brain with electricity.

**American Psychological Association, Psychology Help Center:** https://www.apa.org/helpcenter

Fact sheets and lots of other information about psychological issues that can affect your physical and emotional well-being. Includes a "Find a Psychologist" link to help you locate a licensed psychologist in your area.

**National Alliance on Mental Illness (NAMI):** https://www.nami.org

Information for people with mental health concerns and their family members, including educational material, local resources, and information about local support groups. You can locate a local chapter of NAMI in your area. The organization also operates a helpline at 1-800-950-NAMI (6264), or in a crisis you can text "NAMI" (6264) to 741741.

**National Institute of Neurological Disorders and Stroke, "Mind Your Risks®":** https://www.mindyourrisks.nih.gov/

Useful information from one of the National Institutes of Health geared toward people with high blood pressure, including information about controlling blood pressure in mid-life to help reduce the risk of having a stroke or developing dementia later in life.

**Psychology Today, "Find a Therapist":** https://www.psychologytoday.com/us/therapists

Locate a therapist, psychiatrist, mental health treatment center, or support group in your area, and search by features such as specialization, age, gender, and insurance options.

Norton, P. J., & Antony, M. M. (2021). *The anti-anxiety program: A workbook of proven strategies to overcome worry, panic, and phobias* (2nd ed.). Guilford Press.

User-friendly workbook that teaches you how to use strategies from cognitive behavioral therapy to manage anxiety.

Greenberger, D., & Padesky, C. A. (2015). *Mind over mood: Change how you feel by changing the way you think* (2nd ed.). Guilford Press.

Another user-friendly workbook based on cognitive behavioral therapy, with tools to help you overcome depression, anxiety, anger, guilt, and shame.

Zuckoff, A., & Gorscak, B. (2015). *Finding your way to change: How the power of motivational interviewing can reveal what you want and help you get there.* Guilford Press.

Real examples and practical tools for you to learn how to use principles from motivational interviewing to develop and start your own personal change plan.

Moore, B. A. (2014). *Taking control of anxiety: Small steps for getting the best of worry, stress, and fear.* American Psychological Association. https://www.apa.org/pubs/books/4441023

Concise how-to book that gives case examples and practical techniques to help you manage anxiety.

**Library of Congress, National Library Service for the Blind and Print Disabled, Resources for Senior Citizens and Their Families:** https://www.loc.gov/nls/resources/general-resources-on-disabilities/resources-senior-citizens-families/#_work

This site was designed for people with vision impairment, but it lists dozens of very useful websites related to health care for anyone, including financial resources to assist with health care costs and resources for caregivers.

**U.S. Health Resources and Services Administration, "Find a Health Center":** https://findahealthcenter.hrsa.gov/

Directory of health centers that provide health care on a sliding scale fee based on your income so that it is more affordable. You can search by zip code to find the center closest to you.

**Patient Advocate Foundation, "Finding Care When Uninsured":** https://www.patientadvocate.org/explore-our-resources/getting-care-while-uninsured/finding-care-when-uninsured/

Ideas for finding affordable care for the uninsured and under-insured. The Patient Advocate Foundation main website (https://www.patientadvocate.org) offers other valuable resources, such as information about available financial aid funds and a copayment relief program.

## SELECTED REFERENCES

Alexopoulos, G. S. (2019). Mechanisms and treatment of late-life depression. *Translational Psychiatry, 9*(1), Article 188. https://doi.org/10.1038/s41398-019-0514-6

Alonso-Lana, S., Marquie, M., Ruiz, A., & Boada, M. (2020). Cognitive and neuropsychiatric manifestations of COVID-19 and effects on elderly individuals with dementia. *Frontiers in Aging Neuroscience, 12*, 588872. https://doi.org/10.3389/fnagi.2020.588872

Besser, L., Galvin, J. E., Rodriguez, D., Seeman, T., Kukull, W., Rapp, S. R., & Smith, J. (2019). Associations between neighborhood built environment and cognition vary by apolipoprotein E genotype: Multi-Ethnic Study of Atherosclerosis. *Health Place*, *60*, 102188. https://doi.org/10.1016/j.healthplace.2019.102188

Duric, V., Clayton, S., Leong, M. L., & Yuan, L. L. (2016). Comorbidity factors and brain mechanisms linking chronic stress and systemic illness. *Neural Plasticity*, *2016*, 5460732. https://doi.org/10.1155/2016/5460732

Erickson, K. I., Creswell, J. D., Verstynen, T. D., & Gianaros, P. J. (2014). Health neuroscience: Defining a new field. *Current Directions in Psychological Science*, *23*(6), 446–453. https://doi.org/10.1177/0963721414549350

Forester, B. P., & Gatchel, J. R. (2014). Medical co-morbidity, brain disease, and the future of geriatric psychiatry. *American Journal of Geriatric Psychiatry*, *22*(11), 1061–1065. https://doi.org/10.1016/j.jagp.2014.08.007

Forte, G., & Casagrande, M. (2020). Effects of blood pressure on cognitive performance in aging: A systematic review. *Brain Sciences*, *10*(12). https://doi.org/10.3390/brainsci10120919

Golub, J. S., Brickman, A. M., Ciarleglio, A. J., Schupf, N., & Luchsinger, J. A. (2020). Association of subclinical hearing loss with cognitive performance. *JAMA Otolaryngology–Head & Neck Surgery*, *146*(1), 57–67. https://doi.org/10.1001/jamaoto.2019.3375

Gopalkrishnan, N. (2018). Cultural diversity and mental health: Considerations for policy and practice. *Frontiers in Public Health*, *6*, 179. https://doi.org/10.3389/fpubh.2018.00179

Hooker, S., Punjabi, A., Justesen, K., Boyle, L., & Sherman, M. D. (2018). Encouraging health behavior change: Eight evidence-based strategies. *Family Practice Management*, *25*(2), 31–36. https://www.ncbi.nlm.nih.gov/pubmed/29537244

Lamar, M., Wilson, R. S., Yu, L., James, B. D., Stewart, C. C., Bennett, D. A., & Boyle, P. A. (2019). Associations of literacy with diabetes indicators in older adults. *Journal of Epidemiology and Community Health*, *73*(3), 250–255. https://doi.org/10.1136/jech-2018-210977

McLaren, M. E., Szymkowicz, S. M., O'Shea, A., Woods, A. J., Anton, S. D., & Dotson, V. M. (2017). Vertex-wise examination of depressive symptom dimensions and brain volumes in older adults. *Psychiatry*

*Research: Neuroimaging, 260,* 70–75. https://doi.org/10.1016/j.pscychresns.2016.12.008

Opel, N., Goltermann, J., Hermesdorf, M., Berger, K., Baune, B. T., & Dannlowski, U. (2020). Cross-disorder analysis of brain structural abnormalities in six major psychiatric disorders: A secondary analysis of mega- and meta-analytical findings from the ENIGMA consortium. *Biological Psychiatry, 88*(9), 678–686. https://doi.org/10.1016/j.biopsych.2020.04.027

Pallanti, S., Grassi, E., Makris, N., Gasic, G. P., & Hollander, E. (2020). Neurocovid-19: A clinical neuroscience-based approach to reduce SARS-CoV-2 related mental health sequelae. *Journal of Psychiatric Research, 130,* 215–217. https://doi.org/10.1016/j.jpsychires.2020.08.008

Sharma, R. K., Chern, A., & Golub, J. S. (2021). Age-related hearing loss and the development of cognitive impairment and late-life depression: A scoping overview. *Seminars in Hearing, 42*(1), 10–25. https://doi.org/10.1055/s-0041-1725997

Szcześniak, D., Gladka, A., Misiak, B., Cyran, A., & Rymaszewska, J. (2021). The SARS-CoV-2 and mental health: From biological mechanisms to social consequences. *Progress in Neuro-Psychopharmacology & Biological Psychiatry, 104,* 110046. https://doi.org/10.1016/j.pnpbp.2020.110046

# CHAPTER 8

# PUT IT ALL TOGETHER: START YOUR JOURNEY TO A HEALTHIER BRAIN

"Each of us has that right, that possibility, to invent ourselves daily." This quote, from the late poet, author, and activist Maya Angelou, applies to many facets of life, including our pursuit of a healthier brain. Each day, we can create a healthier version of ourselves by making choices that boost the health of our brain. Our brains are essential to every aspect of life, so when we maintain healthy brains we give ourselves the best chance not just to live, but to live well. Let's review what we can do throughout our lives to achieve and keep healthy brains.

## KEYS TO A HEALTHY BRAIN

Science tells us that people who lead healthy lifestyles are more likely to maintain healthy brains, ones that perform at peak levels. This book summarizes the science-based tools that can help you maximize the health of your brain. You learned that staying physically, mentally, and socially active; getting good nutrition and good sleep; and treating physical and mental health conditions are the healthy behaviors that currently have the most consistent scientific evidence for supporting a healthy brain.

## Physical Activity

Staying physically active is one of the best things you can do to maintain a healthy brain. Research studies show that there is a link between physical fitness and different markers of brain health, such as the size of certain parts of the brain, communication between brain cells, and cognitive functioning. Even stronger evidence comes from clinical trials that randomly assign people to an exercise group or a control group of people who either do not exercise at all or do exercises of lower intensity, such as stretching. Clinical trials show the brain changes for the better in people who start exercising, and their memory and cognitive abilities improve, too. Physical activity can also minimize the decline in memory and other cognitive skills that usually happens as we get older, and it can decrease our risk for Alzheimer's disease and other types of dementia.

Aim for including both aerobic activities and muscle building, or resistance, exercises in your physical activity plan. Aerobic activities should include at least 150 minutes per week of moderate intensity exercises or at least 75 minutes per week of vigorous intensity exercises. Do resistance exercises that include all major muscle groups at least twice each week.

As you plan for a physically active life, remember:

- Even 10-minute bouts of activity can help you reach your weekly goal.
- To stay motivated, pick activities that you enjoy, keep variety in your activities, and, when possible, include a partner or exercise group.
- Consult your doctor or an exercise specialist before starting an exercise program if you have any major health concerns or have not been physically active before now.

- Plan for your physical activities the way you would any other important appointment or weekly activity. Make it a priority and think of ways to overcome obstacles that arise.
- Make it fun! You'll stick to a physically active lifestyle if the activities feel less like work and more like something to enjoy!

## Mental Activity

The adage "Use it or lose it" holds true when it comes to our brains. Science tells us that being mentally active is an important key to lifelong brain health. People who are highly educated, and people who have jobs that require continual learning, problem solving, or critical thinking tend to develop complex and efficient brains. As they grow older, this allows them to maintain their memory and cognitive abilities longer than people who have not had as much mental stimulation, even if they experience common age-related changes in the brain, such as a decrease in the size of different brain regions. This means mental stimulation early in life can help us compensate for some of the effects of aging on the brain. But what you do later in life matters, too. Research studies show that middle-age and older adults who keep their minds active—for example, by starting a stimulating hobby or learning a new skill—can boost their cognitive functioning and even increase the size of brain structures that are important for healthy cognitive functioning, such as the hippocampus and parts of the frontal lobes. And mental activity is one of the ways we can reduce our risk for dementia or slow down memory and cognitive decline if we already have dementia.

As you plan for a mentally active life, remember:

- Think novelty. Focus on adding new activities to your life that engage your brain, challenge you, and are enjoyable.

- Embrace mental challenges. A little bit of strain goes a long way in boosting the health of your brain.
- Ditch the commercially available brain games, such as the ones offered online. There is little scientific evidence that brain games have any substantial benefit on brain health. But if you are concerned about your memory or other cognitive skills, you can ask a neuropsychologist about cognitive training or cognitive rehabilitation; a formal training program with a professional might help.
- Consider activities that include a physical component or a social component. For example, gardening requires planning, attention, and memory, but it is also a good way to introduce more physical activity into your life.
- Let go of stereotypes about aging. You can stay mentally engaged regardless of your age, history, or cognitive abilities.

## Social Activity

We are social creatures by nature, so it is not surprising that we need to stay socially connected to optimize our health and well-being. People who are socially engaged—who interact with others, plan activities with others, and maintain meaningful social relationships— tend to maintain their cognitive skills throughout life and may even be able to improve cognitive functioning and reverse declines in the size of different parts of the brain. Social engagement promotes a sense of well-being and boosts mood, which can make it an effective treatment or prevention strategy for depression. One reason for this link might be that social engagement promotes the health of parts of the brain linked to depression. On the other hand, social isolation can lead to loneliness. Loneliness is linked to cognitive decline and changes in the structure and function of the brain, including the buildup of brain markers of Alzheimer's disease.

As you plan for a socially active life, remember:

- Try to increase your social connections, but be true to yourself. Not everyone desires the same type or amount of social connection.
- Interact regularly with a circle of friends and family with whom you can exchange ideas, thoughts, and concerns. Seek a variety of types of engagement, such as family and cultural events, religious activities, and volunteering.
- Studies show a link between having a sense of purpose and having a healthy brain, so try to add purpose and meaning to your social activities (e.g., by volunteering).
- Remain flexible and try to be creative as you develop a socially active lifestyle. Consider making use of technology in addition to seeing others in person, as well as interacting with animals.
- Try to engage in activities that combine social activity with exercise or a mental challenge, such as playing board games with family members or exercising with a friend.

## Good Nutrition

Despite the confusing and sometimes-contradictory information we hear about what we should or shouldn't eat, research overall supports the idea that dietary patterns are important for maintaining a healthy brain. When you think about the most helpful dietary pattern, think "What's good for the heart is good for the brain." Science tells us that people who follow heart-healthy diets, such as the Mediterranean-style diet, DASH (Dietary Approaches to Stop Hypertension), and the MIND (Mediterranean–DASH Intervention for Neurodegenerative Delay) diet, have a lower risk of heart disease and stroke, less cognitive decline as they age, and a longer life span. These diets all emphasize fruits, vegetables, whole grains, lean meats and fish, beans, and nuts. In contrast, the traditional high-calorie Western diet, which is loaded with red meat, sugar, saturated fat, salt, and refined grains, is linked to heart problems and other diseases, so limit your intake of those types of food. It is worth noting that dietary research is limited by the fact that we cannot completely control people's diets for extended periods of time, so for the most part researchers must rely on what research volunteers say they eat and drink. This means we can't know for sure that specific dietary patterns directly cause improvements in brain health. But as more and more studies come to the same conclusion, it seems worthwhile to adopt a heart-healthy diet to maintain a healthy brain.

As you develop healthy eating habits, remember:

- Dietary *patterns*, not just specific nutrients, are most important for health and wellness. Instead of making a list of specific foods that you absolutely cannot have, or overindulging on the latest "superfood" you hear about, develop long-term healthy eating habits that include a balanced combination of different types of food and nutrients.
- What works for someone else might not work for you, so think about your own challenges, goals, eating habits, and history. Consider journaling to help gain insight into your eating habits and to develop personal goals that make sense for you.
- Research studies show that dietary supplements do not generally improve brain health, and they can even be unsafe. So, unless your doctor tells you that you have a specific nutritional deficiency that requires supplementation, it's best to get your nutrients from eating a balanced diet rather than relying on supplements.
- Don't try to overhaul your diet or keep an overly restrictive diet. Enjoy your food and make small changes that you can build on.
- Plan ahead for your meals to avoid making last-minute decisions about food, which are usually less healthy decisions.

**Good Sleep**

We need sleep to support the functioning of all of our major body systems. Sleep also helps us maintain cognitive and emotional processes, such as our ability to focus attention, to learn and remember information, to control our emotions, and to feel motivated. When we don't get enough sleep, or when the quality of our sleep is poor, our immune system suffers, which increases the risk for various illnesses. Sleep problems can cause different parts of the brain to shrink and can interrupt the production of new brain cells and the communication between parts of the brain. People with sleep problems tend to have difficulties with their cognitive abilities. Vigilance, our ability to continuously maintain focus on a task for an extended period of time, is especially vulnerable. Sleep is important for clearing out toxins in our brains, including toxins that are linked to Alzheimer's disease so, as you might expect, research shows that sleep problems increase the risk for Alzheimer's disease and other types of dementia.

As you develop healthy sleep habits, remember:

- Aim to get 7 to 8 hours of uninterrupted sleep each night, on average, because studies show this is the sweet spot for the best brain health and physical health.
- One of the keys to good sleep is to have a regular sleep–wake schedule. To keep a consistent schedule, pay attention to the timing of your sleep, such as going to bed and waking up at the same time every day and avoiding daytime naps.
- Improve your chances of getting good, restful sleep by exercising and exposing yourself to light during the day and by disconnecting from electronic devices and practicing relaxation strategies, such as mindfulness meditation, before bed.
- Pay attention to your sleep behavior, such as having a regular bedtime routine. Set up a dark, cool, and quiet physical

environment that is conducive to sleep. Try to avoid heavy meals, alcohol, and caffeine late at night.

- See a physician or psychologist who specializes in sleep disorders if you're not sleeping well and notice warning signs of a sleep disorder, such as trouble functioning during the day because of fatigue, problems controlling your emotions, or snoring loudly. And be sure to consult with your doctor about if and how often you should take sleep medication.

## Physical and Mental Health

Physical health, mental health, and brain health are all connected. Physical and psychological conditions can affect your brain, and brain changes can lead to different physical and psychological conditions. Science tells us that we can achieve a healthier brain by treating medical and mental health disorders. In regard to physical health, it is especially important to prevent or treat medical conditions that affect your body's blood supply. This includes keeping your cholesterol and blood pressure in the healthy range for your age; maintaining a healthy body weight; and avoiding smoking to decrease your risk for heart attack, stroke, and other conditions. Vascular diseases and vascular risk factors can affect the health of your brain, leading to cognitive impairment, dementia, and depression. Mid-life is an especially important time for treating these conditions to prevent problems in later life.

The brain is at the center of mental disorders. Studies show that people with psychological conditions such as depression, anxiety disorders, or schizophrenia have brains that differ in size and functioning compared with people who do not have these conditions. Science often shows us a bidirectional relationship between psychological conditions and brain changes given that each can cause the other. For example, changes in the brain can increase your risk for depression, and the reverse is also true: Depression can cause brain changes. When sadness, anxiety, or other psychological symptoms become severe or start to interfere with your functioning, consider seeing a psychologist or another mental health specialist.

To maintain a healthy brain, take care of your physical and mental health. Remember:

- It is important to be proactive about seeing a health care provider if you have physical or mental health concerns. Don't be afraid to ask questions, and make sure to take notes. Get a second opinion or ask for a referral to a specialist if you need to.
- Be open with your health care providers about how personal circumstances, such as where you live, might get in the way of following up on what they're asking you to do for your health. They can help you find opportunities and resources to overcome those barriers, or they can refer you to another professional who can help you find creative ways to stay as healthy as possible regardless of your physical environment.
- Identify barriers to seeking treatment, such as stigma, limited finances, or transportation, and think of ways to overcome them. Ask your health care provider for guidance if you need to.
- If you have mental health concerns, look for a therapist who you feel comfortable with, and don't give up if things don't work out with the first therapist you try.
- Working on physical and mental health takes time and effort. Take it one step at a time.
- Prevention is the best medicine. All of the lifestyle behaviors you've learned about for maintaining a healthy brain can also help to prevent or treat many medical and psychological conditions.

**Get Moving!**

Do aerobic, muscle-building, and balance exercises each week plus moving throughout your day.

**Engage Your Brain!**

Add new activities to your life that engage your brain, challenge you, and are enjoyable.

**Get Connected!**

Build and maintain a social network that gives you a sense of enjoyment and support.

**Nourish Your Brain!**

Keep a heart-healthy diet. Focus on healthy dietary patterns plus specific nutrients. Plan ahead for meals.

**Sleep Well!**

Aim for 7 to 8 hours of good sleep each night. Exercise and get exposure to light during the day.

**Be Well!**

Take care of your physical health, especially your heart. Get treatment for mental health concerns.

## GET STARTED

In my clinical practice, it is always exciting to help clients get started on their journey to a healthier brain. I love it when, armed with the information I share about lifestyle changes and brain health, they seem motivated to start making changes for the health of their brains. The example comes from a 58-year-old woman who came to see me for a neuropsychological evaluation after noting she was regularly misplacing objects and having problems thinking of words during conversations. Testing showed some mild weaknesses in her memory, but my interview with her revealed a set of treatable factors that could have been causing the problem. She had been under considerable stress for many months, symptoms of depression and anxiety; she was getting only 6 hours of sleep each night, and she had chronic back condition that has been linked to cognitive problems.

together to come up with healthy lifestyle goals that would promote
a healthier brain:

- *Physical activity*: The client was already in the habit of taking
  walks or riding her bicycle two or three times weekly. We talked
  about the American Heart Association's (2018) recommendation to include 2 days of strengthening exercises each week.
  She decided to go back to the weekly power yoga classes she
  had enjoyed in the past as a first step toward her goal of doing
  muscle-building activities 2 days a week.
- *Mental activity and social activity*: Because she mentioned reading as a hobby she has always enjoyed, we made a plan for her
  to join a book club as a way of combining cognitive stimulation with social activity. We were able to find clubs in her local
  area as well as online options.
- *Nutrition*: The client mentioned that during all of the stress she
  had been under for a few months, her eating habits changed.
  She had planned to start a diet to lose the 15 pounds she had
  gained, but after learning about the link between nutrition and
  brain health she set a new goal of establishing healthier long-
  term eating habits rather than trying a short-term diet. Her first
  step was to cut back on high-fat and high-sugar food by having
  dessert once a week instead of every day. She also decided to
  meet with a nutritionist to help her set and achieve long-term
  nutrition goals.
- *Sleep, physical health, and mental health*: To work on improving
  her sleep and reducing her stress, depression, anxiety, and
  chronic pain, the client restarted psychotherapy with a therapist she had seen in the past. She made an appointment with
  her primary care doctor to ask about nonpharmacological
  options for treating her chronic pain that could complement
  psychotherapy.

Notice that in many cases, one change addressed multiple aspects of brain health. Joining a book club was a great way for the client to get more mental activity as well as social activity, and going to therapy gave her the opportunity to work on sleep, physical health, and mental health. These multipurpose activities can be a great way to get started in your brain health journey.

Let's be honest: It's hard to make big changes in life. And it's even harder to stick to those changes. Think about how packed gyms are each January, and how they clear out by February or March. Estimates vary, but research studies show that as many as 80% of people who make a New Year's resolution fail to meet their resolution by mid-February. And the numbers hover in the same range when it comes to following through on doctors' recommendations for medications or behavioral changes to manage chronic medical conditions such as obesity, diabetes, or high blood pressure.

Angela Bethea-Walsh, the counseling psychologist you were introduced to in Chapter 7, spends much of her time helping people change their habits to establish healthier lifestyles. Issues such as depression, anxiety, and substance abuse that prompt her clients to seek mental health treatment are often accompanied by insomnia, emotional eating, and other unhealthy behaviors that in turn contribute to their mental health problems. Bethea-Walsh uses a counseling approach called *motivational interviewing* to help her clients find the internal motivation they need to change the behaviors that are keeping them from making healthier choices. She offered some suggestions for how to get started in your journey to a healthier brain.

Similar to other experts I talked to for this book, Bethea-Walsh emphasized the importance of breaking down goals into small, achievable steps. She pointed out that we are more likely to feel motivated to make changes if we are confident that we can reach our goals, so setting realistic goals is really important. You might feel overwhelmed if you try to take on all of the brain-healthy behaviors you've learned about at once. Even if you choose to focus on one of the things we learned—say, increasing your physical activity—it can still be intimidating if you try to quickly switch from getting little exercise at all to meeting expert recommendations for physical activity. Instead, prioritize one or two healthy behaviors to focus on first, and then set a goal for taking one step to get started. Make sure your goals are specific, not vague. As an example, you might choose to start off by working on increasing your physical activity and improving your sleep. What can you choose as your one, specific step toward each of those behaviors? To get more physical activity, you might decide to take an after-dinner walk with your spouse twice a week. To improve your sleep, you might download a mindfulness meditation app for your phone and set a goal of practicing for 10 minutes each day.

Give yourself time to make your new behaviors a habit. It might take a few weeks, or even a few months, but that's a start. Then take the next step. Continuing with the physical activity and sleep example, this might mean stepping up the intensity of your walks or adding in a day of strength training, and cutting out your afternoon naps. Or you might decide to continue what you've already been doing as far as exercising and sleep, but add in a nutrition goal, such as cutting back on the salt in your diet. Either way, take another small step, make it a habit, and then take the next step. Keep doing this until you reach the goals you set for yourself. Set short- and long-term goals. Your short-term goals are the small steps you're taking to ultimately get to your long-term goal. This is a gradual process to develop lifelong habits that will help you achieve a healthy brain. It will not happen overnight, so don't put pressure on yourself by setting unrealistic goals.

Part of being realistic as you start on your journey is knowing that you will not always meet your short-term goals, and that is OK. I like the way Bethea-Walsh put it—she advised that we "reset the button" when we don't reach our goals, rather than punishing ourselves. Life happens, emergencies happen, and sometimes our motivation just isn't there. If you set a goal for the week and you don't quite meet your goal, reset the button and try again the next week. Have self-compassion, because giving in to feelings of guilt or embarrassment after trying and falling short will only lead to more negative feelings, such as depression and anxiety, and those feelings are counterproductive to change. Research shows that long-lasting change is more likely to happen when it is self-motivated and rooted in positive thinking, not when driven by fear or regret.

Experts also agree that it's important to have practical ways of reaching your goals. As we have done throughout this book, think about barriers ahead of time and try to think of solutions to overcome them. Know what your resources are. For example, it might not be practical to set a goal of learning to play a new musical instrument as a means of increasing your mental activity if you don't have access to your instrument of choice. It might be more practical to take an online music appreciation class to act on your love of music.

## CARRY ON

My goal for this book is to empower you with science-based facts and practical tools to achieve and maintain a healthy brain. The brain—this fascinating, complex, 3-pound structure that controls every function of our body—enables us to live well *if* we take care of it. By keeping our brain as healthy as possible, we can optimize our cognitive abilities, our mental health, and our physical functioning at any age. In the face of the threat of Alzheimer's disease and other types of dementia as we grow older, good brain health offers the possibility of slowing down or maybe even preventing these feared conditions.

As you proceed in your journey to achieve the healthiest brain possible, remember your reasons for making changes to your life. Science tells us that our lifestyle choices can change our brains for the better or for the worse, and you have chosen to improve your brain health to live your fullest life now and to age better. Embrace this as a lifelong process, as something to work on little by little every day. Don't give up when your motivation wavers or when you don't reach a goal you set. Each day is a new day to start again. Keep going. Invent yourself daily.

## RESOURCES AND SUGGESTED READINGS

**CerebroFit Integrated Brain Health:** https://cerebrofit.org/
Website for my company. We offer services to help you achieve and maintain a healthy brain, such as personal training, nutrition consultations, health coaching, psychotherapy, and neuropsychological assessment. Services are available through telehealth and in person in the Atlanta, Georgia, area. You can sign up for our blog to hear about the latest research related to keeping a healthy brain!

**Alzheimer's Association:** https://www.alz.org/
Educational information and resources related to Alzheimer's disease, other types of dementia, and cognitive aging in people without dementia. Includes lots of information for caregivers as well as local resources.

**AARP, "Staying Sharp®":** https://stayingsharp.aarp.org/
Information about how to join the Staying Sharp program, which gives step-by-step guidance for living a lifestyle that promotes brain health. Based on the Global Council on Brain Health.

**Eldercare Locator:** https://www.eldercare.acl.gov/
Educational information and services for seniors and caregivers. Connect to organizations in your local area by zip code or city and state.

## SELECTED REFERENCE

American Heart Association. (2018, April 18). *American Heart Association recommendations for physical activity in adults and kids.* https://www.heart.org/en/healthy-living/fitness/fitness-basics/aha-recs-for-physical-activity-in-adults

# INDEX

for sleep, 154–163, 201–202
for social activity, 105–115, 199
Plaque, atherosclerotic, 172
Polysomnography, 147
Powell, T., 92
Prefrontal cortex, 103–104, 174
Prevagen, 127–128
Preventing health problems, 186, 188
Prioritization, of healthy food, 133
Problem solving, for mental stimulation, 71
Processing speed, 102
Psychiatric disorders, social behavior and, 98
Psychiatric nurses, 181
Psychiatrists, 180
Psychological diagnosis, in neuropsychological evaluations, 8
Psychological eating cues, 130
Psychologist Locator (website), 182
Psychologists, 180
Psychology Help Center, 190
*Psychology Today*, 14, 191
Psychotherapy, 180, 181, 187
Public transportation, 63, 187
Purpose
after retirement, 75
mental activities, 88
in social activities, 107–110, 113

Racial disparities
in access to mental health treatment, 186
in health risks, 176
Randolph, J., 14–15
"The Real Deal on Brain Health Supplements" (Global Council on Brain Health), 141
Reasoning skills, 77, 102
Reasoning training, 78
Rebekah Circle, 105
Reductionist approach in nutritional science, 122
Referrals, to therapists, 183

Relationships, influence of, on eating habits, 132
Relaxation response, 160
*The Relaxation Response* (Benson & Klipper), 160
Relaxation strategies, 160–161
Relocation, social engagement and, 109
Replicability, of research, 25, 80
Research
characteristics of, 25–28
on mental activities, 70–81
on nutrition, 122–128
on physical activity, 36–47
on sleep, 146–154
on social activities, 98–105
types of, 26–28
on wellness, 170–177
Resistance training, 14, 49, 52, 54, 55, 59, 63
Resources for Senior Citizens and Their Families (website), 192
Resting state (of brain), 38
Restricted sleep, 149
Retirement, 74–75, 109
"Rewiring the brain" with exercise, 40
Rush Medical Center, 172
Rush University, 124

Safety, in physical activity, 54–56
Scheduling physical activity, 49, 53, 55
Science-based information, reputable sources of, 22–25
Scientific advisory boards, 80–81
Scientific research, 25–28
Seated exercises, 63
Self-consciousness, 63
Sense about Science, 29
Senses, brain's support of, 10–11
Sensory changes, 173–174
7 Best Sleep Apps for iPhone and Android (website), 165
"7 Ways to Promote Brain Health During a Pandemic" (Randolph), 14–15

# ABOUT THE AUTHOR

**Vonetta M. Dotson, PhD,** is a neuropsychologist, author, and speaker. She has spent over 20 years teaching, providing clinical care, and conducting research related to brain health and aging. She is founder and president of the Atlanta-based company CerebroFit Integrated Brain Health (https://cerebrofit.org/), which offers neuropsychological assessments and services such as personal training and nutrition consultations to support a healthy brain. She is also an associate professor of psychology and gerontology at Georgia State University, Senior Project Scientist at NASA, and a Fellow of the American Psychological Association's Society for Clinical Neuropsychology. She completed her doctoral training in clinical psychology at the University of Florida in 2006 with a specialization in neuropsychology and a certificate in gerontology, and she completed her postdoctoral training at the National Institute on Aging. In both her personal and professional life, Dr. Dotson is passionate about the power of exercise and other healthy behaviors to protect brain health, boost mental skills, and treat mental illnesses such as depression.